Foot and
Lower Extremity
Anatomy to Color
and Study

Foot and Lower Extremity Anatomy to Color and Study

Ray Poritsky, Ph.D. Emeritus
Department of Anatomy
Case Western Reserve University
Cleveland, Ohio

HANLEY & BELFUS, INC., Medical Publishers/Philadelphia

Publisher: HANLEY & BELFUS, INC.
               Medical Publishers
               210 South 13th Street
               Philadelphia, PA 19107
               215/546-7293, 800/962-1892
               www.hanleyandbelfus.com

Library of Congress Cataloging-in-Publication Data

Foot and lower extremity anatomy to color and study/Ray Poritsky.
        p. ; cm.
     ISBN 1-56053-481-8 (alk. paper)
     1. Leg—Anatomy—Atlases. 2. Foot—Anatomy—Atlases. 3. Coloring books. I.
Poritsky, Raphael.
     [DNLM: 1. Foot—anatomy & histology—Atlases. 2. Leg—anatomy &
histology—Atlases. WE 17 F687 2001]
     QM549 .F66 2001
     611'.98'0222—dc21   00-054273

Foot and Lower Extremity Anatomy to Color and Study   ISBN 1-56053-481-8

Last digit is the print number: 9 8 7 6 5 4 3 2 1

Contents

Preface

This book is designed to help students learn the complex anatomy of the lower extremity. It also serves as a comprehensive review for students at the completion of their gross anatomy course. The various muscles, nerves, and blood vessels of the lower limb are depicted in bold black and white drawings for the reader to label and color. The reader may wish to simply identify each structure by its name and not color it. The use of color, however, will help delineate the structure in question, such as a muscle, or in the case of a vessel or nerve, adding color will more clearly reveal its path and distribution. Indeed, labelling each structure and adding color calls upon the reader to play a more active role rather than simply reading about anatomy in a book. I hope that this book will make it easier to master the anatomy of the lower limb. I also welcome suggestions and comments from readers.

I have used many of the beautiful pen and ink drawings by Eycleshymer and Jones published in 1925 in their classic *Hand Atlas of Clinical Anatomy*. These clear concise drawings were an outgrowth of their very popular *Manual of Surgical Anatomy* prepared for the army and navy medical corps during the First World War. I have updated the Latin names and relabelled them with current anatomical terms. In most of their drawings, I have added new leaders (connecting lines). In a few cases, I have modified the Eycleshymer and Jones drawings to include present day anatomical knowledge.

I have included a few etymological cartoons that I hope will afford a little levity in what can be, at times, a challenging subject, the anatomy of the upper limb. The knowledge of how each part of the body got its name is actually quite interesting and often makes it easier to remember that particular anatomy.

Color pencils at the ready! Go and Good Luck!

RAY PORITSKY, PH.D.
Cleveland, Ohio

Acknowledgments

Additional figures were drawn by Cheryl Owens. Most of the illustrations are reworked and updated figures from Eycleshymer and Jones: *Hand Atlas of Clinical Anatomy*, Lea & Febiger, 1925. Atlases and texts that I used to draw figures for this book are: Wolf-Heidegger: *Atlas of Systemic Human Anatomy*, Hafner, 1962; Spalteholz and Spanner: *Atlas of Human Anatomy, 16th ed.*, F.A. Davis, 1961; Hollinshead and Rosse: *Textbook of Anatomy, 4th ed.*, Harper and Row, 1985; Clemente: *A Regional Atlas of the Human Body, 3rd ed.*, Urban & Schwarzenberg, 1987; Töndury, *Angewandte und Topographische Anatomie*, Fretz & Wasmuth, 1949; Williams (ed): *Gray's Anatomy, 38th British ed.*, Churchill Livingstone, 1995; Netter: *The Ciba Collection of Medical Illustrations*, Ciba Pharmaceutical Company, 1959.

I wish to thank my publisher and editor, Linda Belfus, for her generous support and encouragement for this book and to her most helpful staff at Hanley and Belfus in Philadelphia, especially Denise Roslonski.

I thank and warmly dedicate this book to my wife Connie.

1 Bones of the lower extremity

Including coxal bone

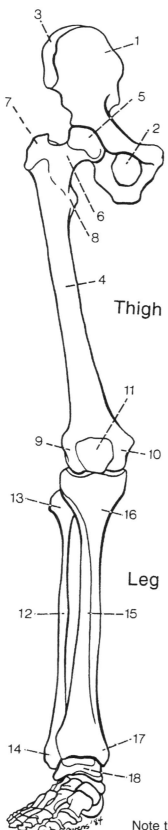

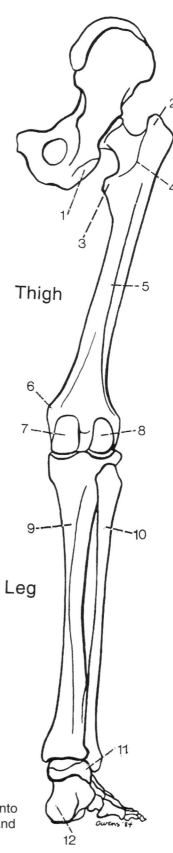

◀ Right leg Anterior view

Color and label

1 Coxal bone (hip bone)
2 Obturator foramen
3 Iliac crest
4 Femur
5 Head of femur
6 Neck of femur
7 Greater trochanter
8 Lesser trochanter
9 Lateral epicondyle
10 Medial epicondyle
11 Patella
12 Fibula
13 Head of fibula
14 Lateral malleolus
15 Tibia
16 Tibial tuberosity
17 Medial malleolus
18 Talus

Right leg Posterior view ▶

1 Ischial tuberosity
2 Greater trochanter
3 Lesser trochanter
4 Intertrochanteric crest
5 Linea aspera
6 Adductor tubercle
7 Medial condyle
8 Lateral condyle
9 Tibia
10 Fibula
11 Talus
12 Calcaneus

Note that in anatomy the lower extremity is divided into an upper **thigh** extending from the hip to the knee and lower **leg** that extends from the knee to the ankle.

Anterior view

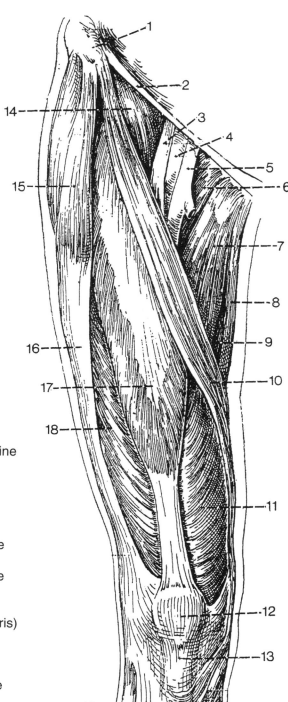

Color and label

1 Anterior superior iliac spine
2 Inguinal ligament
3 Femoral nerve
4 Femoral artery
5 Femoral vein
6 Pectineus muscle
7 Adductor magnus muscle
8 Gracilis muscle
9 Adductor magnus muscle
10 Sartorius muscle
11 Vastus medialis muscle
   (part of quadriceps femoris)
12 Patella (knee cap)
13 Patellar ligament
14 Iliopsoas muscle
15 Tensor fascia lata muscle
16 Iliotibial tract
17 Rectus femoris muscle
   (part of quadriceps femoris)
18 Vastus lateralis
   (part of quadriceps femoris)
19 Tibial tuberosity
   (insertion of quadriceps femoris)

Eycleshymer and Jones

Muscle (etymological cartoon)

To the ancient Romans, contracted muscle looked like small mice running under the skin, so they named the fleshy red bundles of the body musculi, which means "little mice," musculus being the diminutive of mus, mouse.

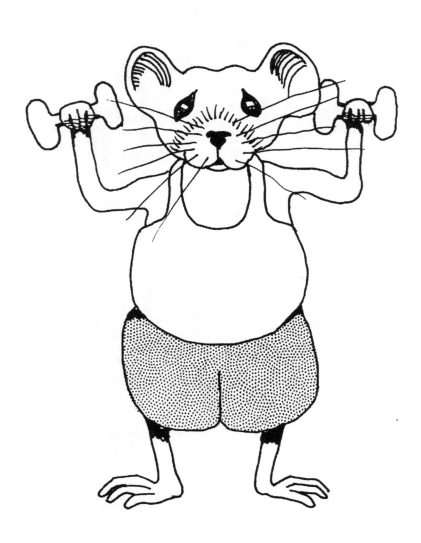

Lateral view

Color and label

1 Sartorius muscle
2 Tensor facia lata muscle
3 Greater trochanter (of femur; palpable beneath the skin)
4 Rectus femoris muscle
5 Iliotibial tract
6 Vastus lateralis muscle
7 Gluteus maximus muscle
8 Biceps femoris muscle (long head)
9 Biceps femoris muscle (short head)
10 Semimembranosus muscle
11 Tendon of biceps femoris
12 Gastrocnemius muscle (lateral head)
13 Soleus muscle
14 Patella
15 Insertion of biceps femoris on head of fibula
16 Tibial tuberosity

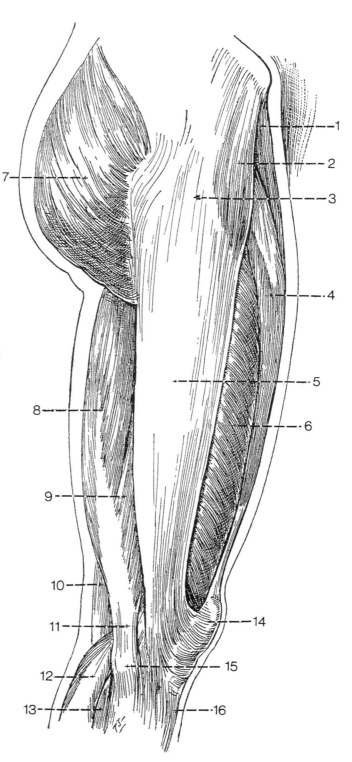

Eycleshymer and Jones

4 Superficial muscles of the right thigh

Posterior view

Color and label

1 Gluteus medius muscle
  (under gluteal fascia)
2 Gluteus maximus muscle
3 Greater trochanter of femur
4 Adductor magnus muscle
5 Iliotibial tract
6 Semimembranosus muscle
7 Biceps femoris muscle
8 Semitendinosus muscle
9 Semimembranosus muscle
10 Gracilis muscle
11 Sartorius muscle
12 Plantaris muscle
13 Tendon of biceps femoris
14 Gastrocnemius muscle

Eycleshymer and Jones

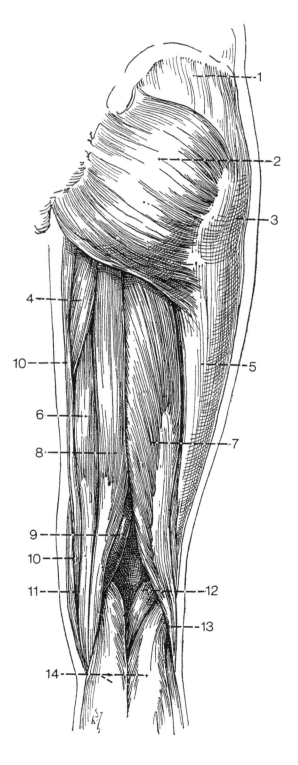

5 Superficial muscles of the leg

Anterior aspect

Color and label

1 Vastus medialis muscle
2 Tibial collateral ligament
3 Medial lemniscus
4 Medial patellar retinaculum
  (cut open to expose medial lemniscus)
5 Sartorius tendon (insertion on tibia)
6 Gastrocnemius muscle
7 Medial surface of tibia
8 Soleus muscle
9 Extensor hallucis longus muscle
10 Tendon of tibialis anterior
11 Medial malleolus
12 Extensor hallucis brevis muscle
13 Tendon of extensor hallucis longus
14 Vastus lateralis muscle
15 Iliotibial tract
16 Patella
17 Fibular collateral ligament
18 Patellar ligament
19 Tibial tuberosity
20 Peroneus longus muscle
21 Tibialis anterior muscle
22 Extensor digitorum longus muscle
23 Peroneus brevis muscle
24 Fibula
25 Superior extensor muscular retinaculum
26 Lateral malleolus
27 Inferior extensor muscular retinaculum
28 Tendon of peroneus tertius
29 Tendons of extensor digitorum

Eycleshymer and Jones

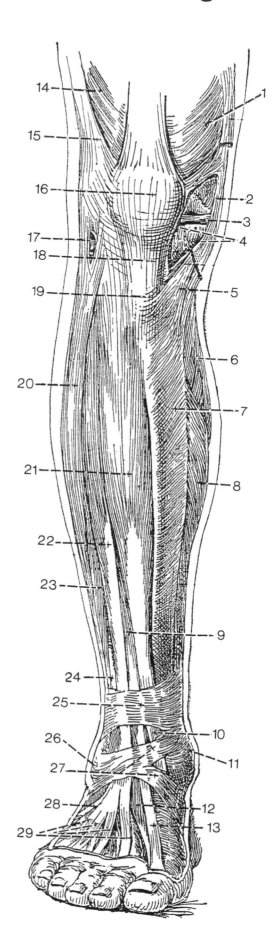

6 Superficial muscles of the right leg

Lateral aspect

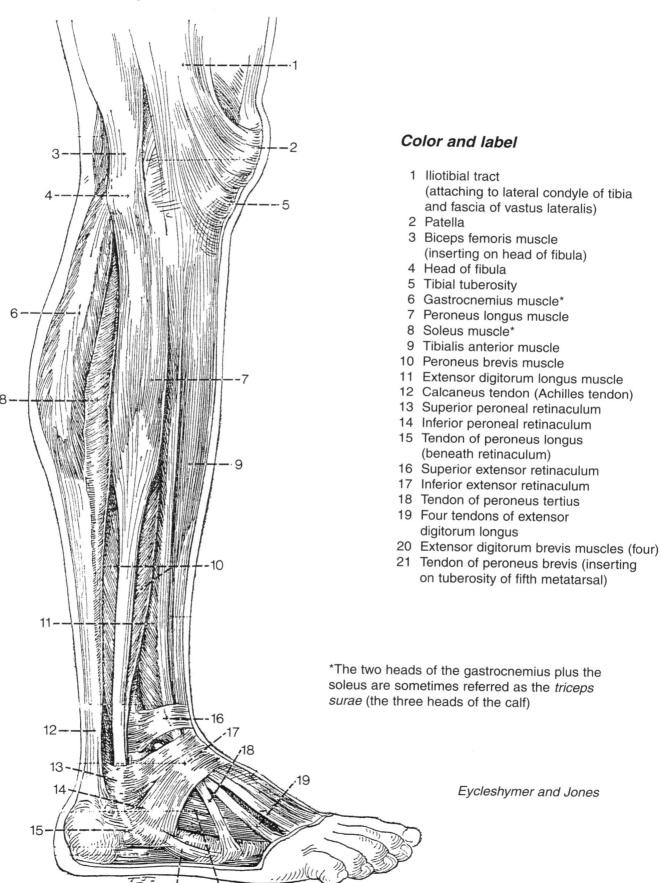

Color and label

1 Iliotibial tract
(attaching to lateral condyle of tibia
and fascia of vastus lateralis)
2 Patella
3 Biceps femoris muscle
(inserting on head of fibula)
4 Head of fibula
5 Tibial tuberosity
6 Gastrocnemius muscle*
7 Peroneus longus muscle
8 Soleus muscle*
9 Tibialis anterior muscle
10 Peroneus brevis muscle
11 Extensor digitorum longus muscle
12 Calcaneus tendon (Achilles tendon)
13 Superior peroneal retinaculum
14 Inferior peroneal retinaculum
15 Tendon of peroneus longus
(beneath retinaculum)
16 Superior extensor retinaculum
17 Inferior extensor retinaculum
18 Tendon of peroneus tertius
19 Four tendons of extensor
digitorum longus
20 Extensor digitorum brevis muscles (four)
21 Tendon of peroneus brevis (inserting
on tuberosity of fifth metatarsal)

*The two heads of the gastrocnemius plus the
soleus are sometimes referred as the *triceps
surae* (the three heads of the calf)

Eycleshymer and Jones

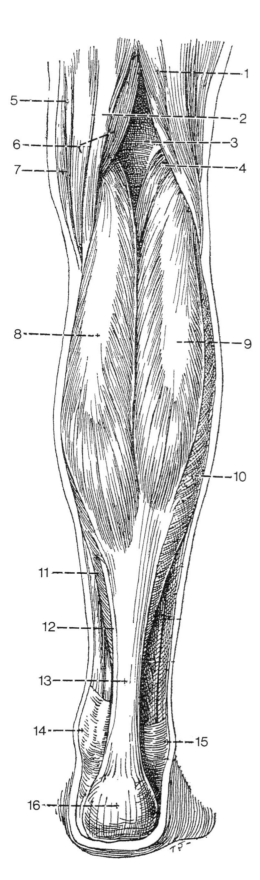

Color and label

1 Biceps femoris muscle
2 Semitendinosus muscle
3 Popliteal fossa
4 Plantaris muscle
5 Gracilis muscle
6 Semimembranosus muscle
7 Sartorius muscle
8 Gastrocnemius muscle (medial head)
9 Gastrocnemius muscle (lateral head)
10 Soleus muscle (deep to gastrocnemius)
11 Soleus muscle (deep to gastrocnemius)
12 Tendon of plantaris muscle (this small
   muscle has a long thin tendon that
   descends with the calcaneal tendon
   and inserts separately on the
   calcaneal tuberosity)
13 Calcaneal tendon (Achilles tendon)
14 Medial malleolus of tibia
15 Lateral malleolus of fibula
16 Calcaneal tuberosity

Eycleshymer and Jones

8 Muscles of medial right leg

1 Gracilis muscle
2 Semimembranosus muscle
3 Semitendinosus muscle
4 Tendon of gracilis
5 Tendon of semimembranosus
6 Semitendinosus tendon
7 Gastrocnemius muscle
   (medial head)
8 Soleus muscle)
9 Flexor digitorum longus muscle
10 Flexor hallucis longus muscle
11 Tibialis posterior tendon
   (synovial sheath)
12 Flexor digitorum longus
   tendon (synovial sheath)
13 Calcaneal tendon
   (Achilles tendon)
14 Flexor hallucis longus
   tendon (synovial sheath)
15 Flexor retinaculum
16 Abductor hallucis muscle
17 Tendon of flexor hallucis
   longus (synovial sheath)
18 Tendon of tibialis anterior
19 Abductor hallucis
20 Sartorius muscle
21 Vastus medialis muscle
22 Patella
23 Patellar ligament
24 Pes anserinus*
25 Tibialis anterior muscle
26 Tibia
27 Medial malleolus
28 Inferior extensor retinaculum
29 Tendon of tibialis anterior
   (synovial sheath)
30 Synovial sheaths of extensor
   digitorum longus tendons
31 Synovial sheath of extensor
   hallucis longus
32 Extensor digitorum
   longus tendons
33 Tendon of extensor
   hallucis longus

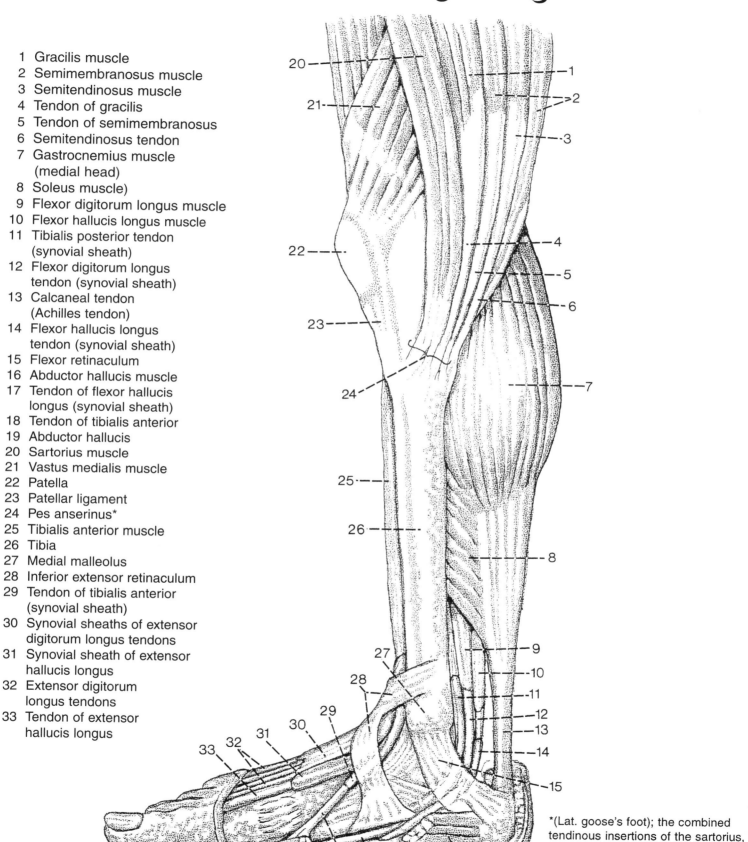

*(Lat. goose's foot); the combined
tendinous insertions of the sartorius,
gracilis, and semitendinosus on the
medial tibia in a manner resembling
the webbed foot of a goose.

Redrawn from Clemente

9 Right coxal bone (innominate bone, hip bone)

Lateral (external) aspect

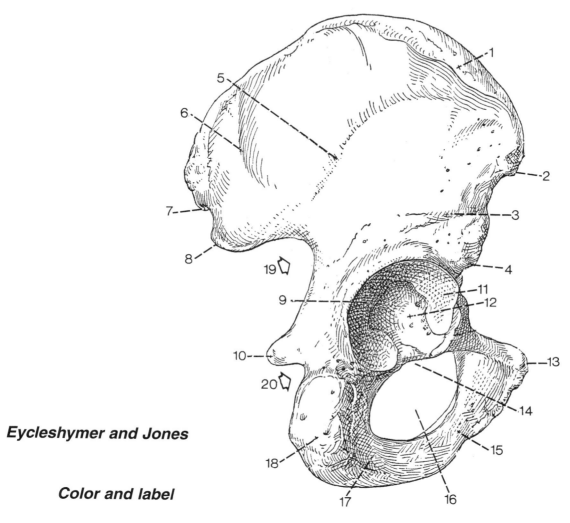

Eycleshymer and Jones

Color and label

1 Crest of the ilium
2 Anterior superior iliac spine
3 Inferior gluteal line
4 Anterior inferior iliac spine
5 Anterior gluteal line
6 Posterior gluteal line
7 Posterior superior iliac spine
8 Posterior inferior iliac spine
9 Acetabulum (socket for the head of the femur)
10 Ischial spine

11 Lunate surface (articular surface)
12 Acetabular fossa (rough non-articular portion above acetabular notch)
13 Pubic tubercle
14 Acetabular notch
15 Inferior pubic ramus
16 Obturator foramen*
17 Ischial ramus
18 Ischial tuberosity
19 Greater sciatic notch
20 Lesser sciatic notch

*The obturator foramen or the "stopped up foramen" (by muscle and membrane) takes its name from the Latin *obturare*, "to stop up"; the blockage, however, is not complete; the small obturator canal allows the passage of the obturator nerve, artery, and vein.

Medial (internal) surface

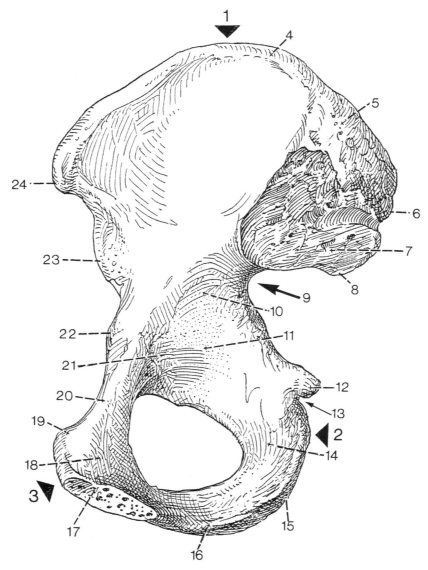

Eycleshymer and Jones

1 Ilium	13 Lesser sciatic notch
2 Ischium	14 Ramus of ischium
3 Pubis	15 Ischial tuberosity
4 Iliac crest	16 Inferior pubic ramus
5 Iliac tuberosity	17 Symphysial surface of pubis;
6 Posterior superior iliac spine	articulates with opposite pubis
7 Auricular surface;	in the pubic symphysis
articulates with sacrum	18 Superior pubic ramus
8 Posterior inferior iliac spine	19 Pubic tubercle
9 Greater sciatic notch	20 Pecten pubis (*pecten*, Latin,
10 Body of ilium	comb, comb-like)
11 Body of pubis	21 Body of pubic bone
12 Spine of the ischium	22 Iliopectineal eminence
(ischial spine)	23 Anterior inferior iliac spine
	24 Anterior superior iliac spine

11 The right femur

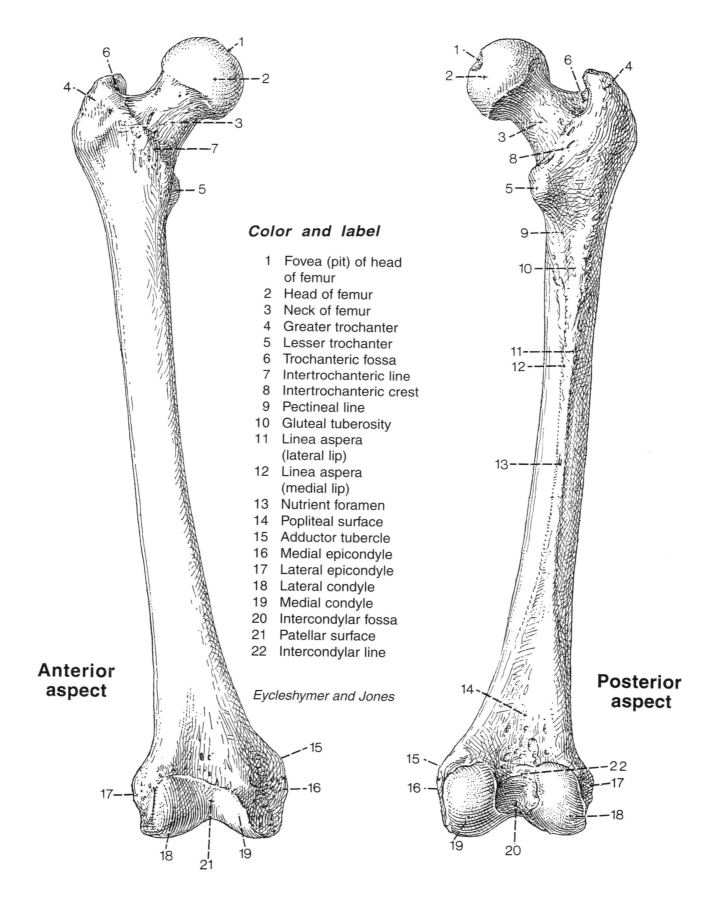

Anterior aspect

Posterior aspect

Color and label

1 Fovea (pit) of head of femur
2 Head of femur
3 Neck of femur
4 Greater trochanter
5 Lesser trochanter
6 Trochanteric fossa
7 Intertrochanteric line
8 Intertrochanteric crest
9 Pectineal line
10 Gluteal tuberosity
11 Linea aspera (lateral lip)
12 Linea aspera (medial lip)
13 Nutrient foramen
14 Popliteal surface
15 Adductor tubercle
16 Medial epicondyle
17 Lateral epicondyle
18 Lateral condyle
19 Medial condyle
20 Intercondylar fossa
21 Patellar surface
22 Intercondylar line

Eycleshymer and Jones

Fibula and Tibia (etymological cartoon)

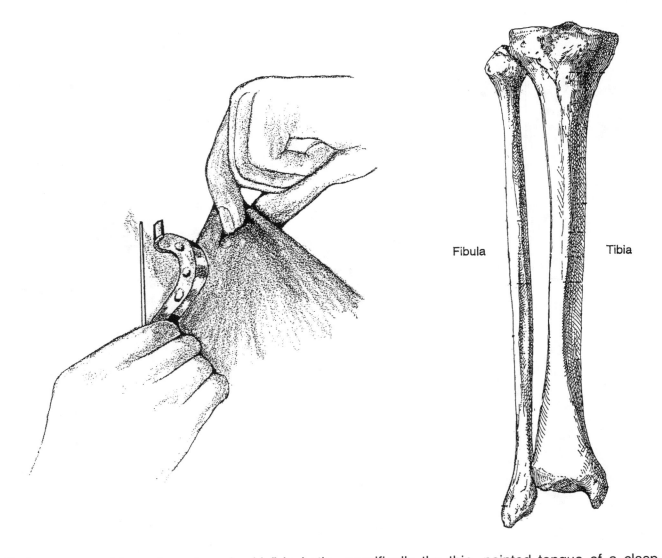

Fibula   Tibia

Fibula means a "clasp, brooch or buckle" in Latin, specifically the thin, pointed tongue of a clasp, as opposed to the much thicker, and often highly ornate, bar of the clasp. Supposedly the Romans thought that the two bones of the lower leg resembled a clasp, with the outer thin fibula suggesting the tongue and the inner thicker tibia suggesting the bar. So they named the thin outer one *fibula*, and the more stout inner one *tibia*. The term *fibula* probably arose from the verb *figo*, "to fix" or "to fasten." The muscles and structures on the outer side of the lower leg that relate to the fibula were named by English-speaking anatomists not **fibular**, as one might expect, but peroneal, from the Greek word for "brooch", *perone*, which is derived from the verb *peiro*, "to pierce". However, anatomists in countries such as Germany and Switzerland preferred to name these lateral muscles, nerves, and blood vessels **fibular**. So depending on where one studies anatomy, one will learn the outer lower leg muscles and related structures as either **fibular** or **peroneal**. As for remembering which bone is the tibia and which is the fibula, the fibula, which is **lateral**, ends with **la** as in **la**teral. The term **tibia** means a "flute" or "pipe" in Latin as well as the shin bone. The ancients probably made flute-like instruments from the shin bones of animals.

12 Right tibia and fibula

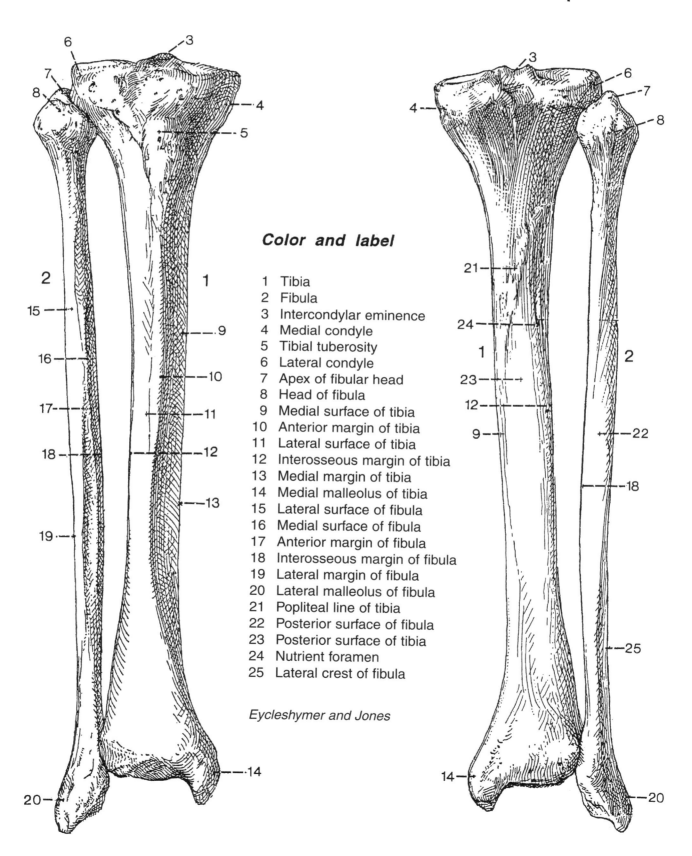

Anterior aspect

6
3
7
8
4
5
2
1
15
9
16
10
17
11
18
12
13
19
14
20

Posterior aspect

3
6
7
8
4
21
24
1
2
23
12
9
22
18
14
25
20

Color and label

1 Tibia
2 Fibula
3 Intercondylar eminence
4 Medial condyle
5 Tibial tuberosity
6 Lateral condyle
7 Apex of fibular head
8 Head of fibula
9 Medial surface of tibia
10 Anterior margin of tibia
11 Lateral surface of tibia
12 Interosseous margin of tibia
13 Medial margin of tibia
14 Medial malleolus of tibia
15 Lateral surface of fibula
16 Medial surface of fibula
17 Anterior margin of fibula
18 Interosseous margin of fibula
19 Lateral margin of fibula
20 Lateral malleolus of fibula
21 Popliteal line of tibia
22 Posterior surface of fibula
23 Posterior surface of tibia
24 Nutrient foramen
25 Lateral crest of fibula

Eycleshymer and Jones

13 Bones of the right foot

Viewed from above

Viewed from below

Eycleshymer and Jones

Color and label

1 Calcaneus
2 Talus
3 Navicular
4 Cuboid
5 Medial cuneiform
6 Intermediate cuneiform
7 Lateral cuneiform
8 Trochlea (Latin, pulley) of talus
9 Lateral process of talus
10 Neck of talus
11 Head of talus
12 First metatarsal
13 Proximal phalanx of big toe (hallux, Latin)
14 Distal phalanx of big toe

15 Tuberosity of fifth metatarsal
16 Calcaneal tuber (Latin, swelling, protuberance)
17 Lateral process of calcaneal tuber
18 Medial process of calcaneal tuber
19 Sustentaculum tali (support of talus) of calcaneus
20 Tuberosity of first metatarsal
21 Sesamoid bones
22 Fifth metatarsal
23 Proximal phalanx of fifth toe
24 Middle phalanx of fifth toe
25 Distal phalanx of fifth toe

14 Lumbar muscles

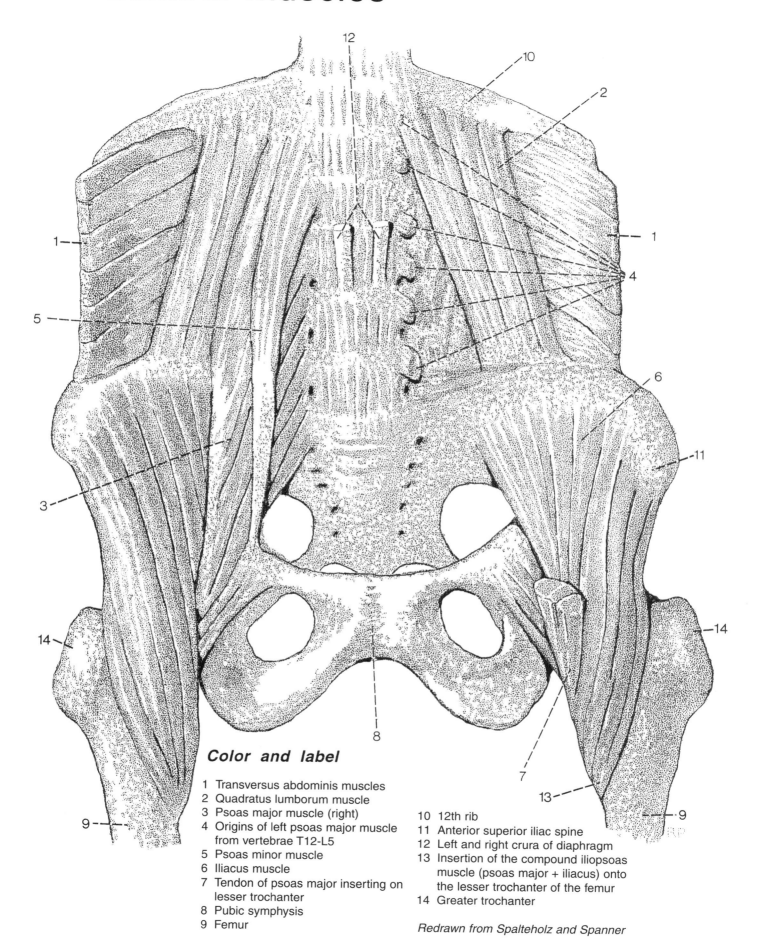

Color and label

1 Transversus abdominis muscles
2 Quadratus lumborum muscle
3 Psoas major muscle (right)
4 Origins of left psoas major muscle from vertebrae T12-L5
5 Psoas minor muscle
6 Iliacus muscle
7 Tendon of psoas major inserting on lesser trochanter
8 Pubic symphysis
9 Femur

10 12th rib
11 Anterior superior iliac spine
12 Left and right crura of diaphragm
13 Insertion of the compound iliopsoas muscle (psoas major + iliacus) onto the lesser trochanter of the femur
14 Greater trochanter

Redrawn from Spalteholz and Spanner

15 Arteries of the right thigh

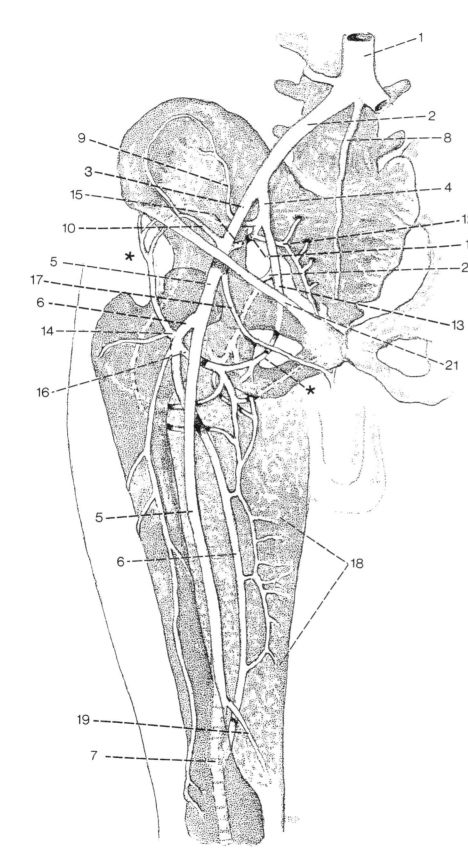

Color and label

1 Abdominal aorta
2 Right common iliac artery
3 External iliac artery
4 Internal iliac artery
5 Femoral artery; the external
  iliac artery becomes the femoral
  artery below the inguinal ligament.
6 Deep femoral artery
7 Popliteal artery (posterior to
  the femur); the femoral artery
  becomes the popliteal artery
  below the adductor hiatus.
  The names of the accompanying
  veins (not shown) undergo similar
  changes.
8 Median sacral artery
9 Iliolumbar artery
10 Deep iliac circumflex artery
11 Superior gluteal artery
12 Lateral sacral artery
13 Obturator artery
14 Lateral femoral circumflex artery
   (*anastamosis between 10 and 14
   is exaggerated in thickness to
   illustrate collateral circulation in
   case of blockage of the upper
   femoral artery)
15 Inferior epigastric artery (cut)
16 Medial femoral circumflex artery
   (*anastamosis between 13 and 16
   is exaggerated in thickness to show
   possible collateral circulation)
17 External pudendal artery
18 Perforating branches of
   deep femoral artery
19 Descending genicular artery
20 Inferior gluteal artery
21 Inguinal artery

Redrawn from Eycleshymer and Jones

Color and label

1 Subcostal nerve (T12)
2 Iliohypogastric nerve
3 Ilioinguinal nerve
4 Anterior scrotal branches
 of ilioinguinal nerve
 (labial in female)
5 Genitofemoral nerve
6 Genital branch of
 genitofemoral nerve
7 Femoral branch of
 genitofemoral nerve
8 Lateral femoral
 cutaneous nerve
9 Obturator nerve; note
 that both the obturator
 and the femoral nerve
 arise from lumbar
 nerves L2, L3, L4.
10 Anterior branch of
 obturator nerve
11 Posterior branch of
 obturator nerve
12 Femoral nerve
13 Saphenous nerve (branch
 of femoral nerve)
14 Muscular branches of the
 femoral nerve; the femoral
 nerve supplies all the muscles
 in the anterior compartment
 of the thigh.
15 Anterior cutaneous branches
 of the femoral nerve
16 Lumbosacral trunk; carries
 fibers from L4 and L5 to
 sacral plexus.
17 Sacral nerves S1-S5
18 Sacral plexus
19 Twelfth rib
20 Right testis
21 Inguinal canal (schematic)

NL1-L5, lumbar nerves
L1-L5, lumbar vertebrae

Redrawn from Spalteholz and Spanner

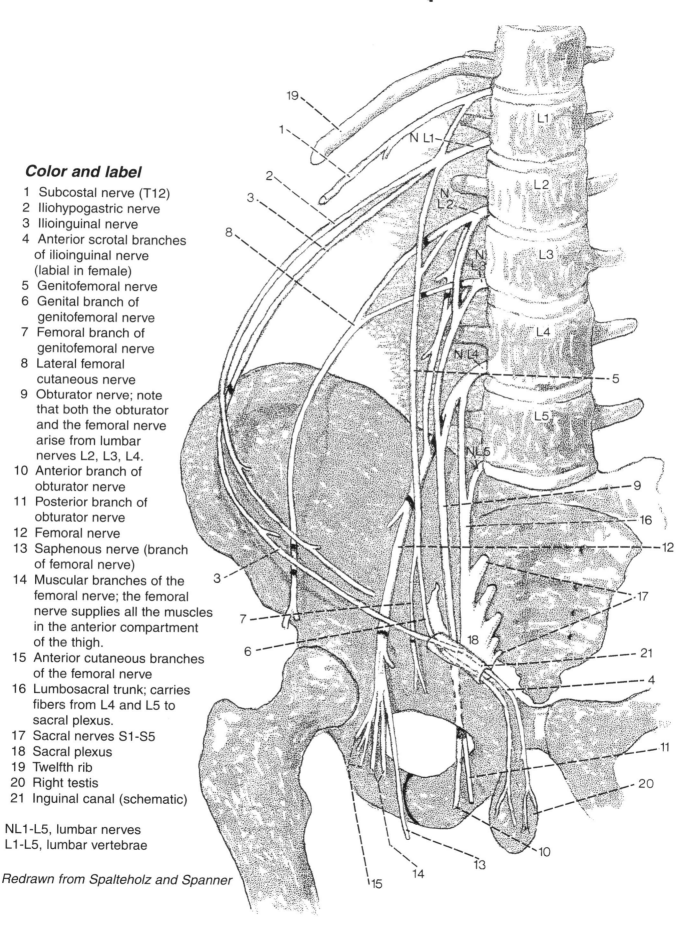

The following muscles are innervated by the femoral nerve except where otherwise indicated. Small portions of these muscles are indicated on the figure's left.

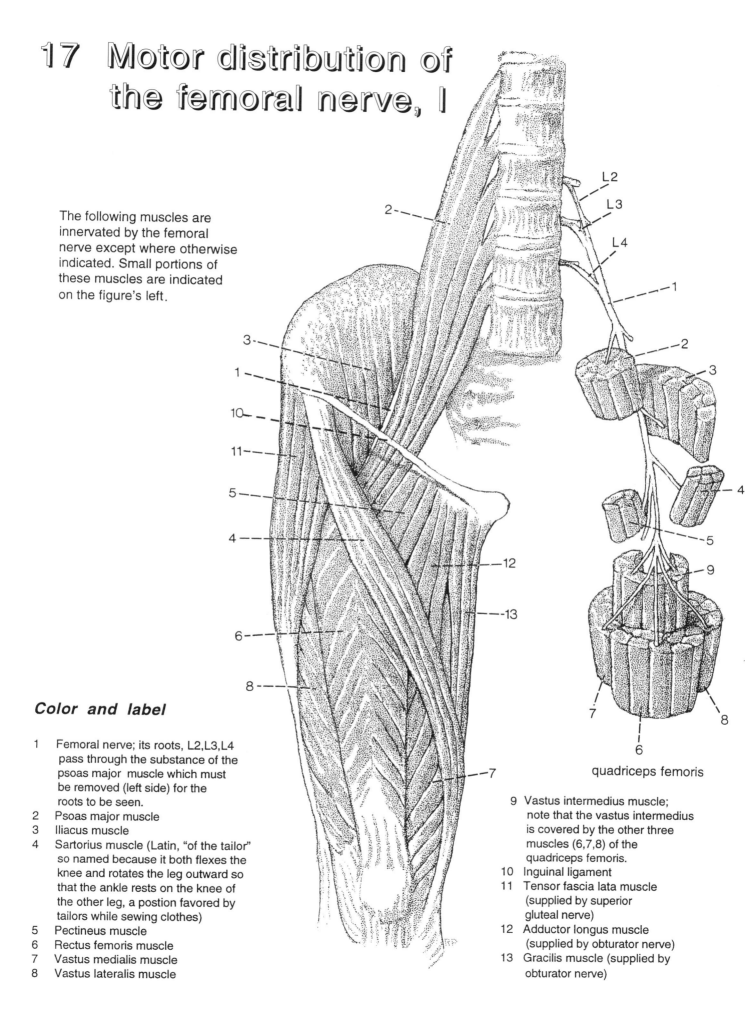

quadriceps femoris

Color and label

1 Femoral nerve; its roots, L2,L3,L4 pass through the substance of the psoas major muscle which must be removed (left side) for the roots to be seen.
2 Psoas major muscle
3 Iliacus muscle
4 Sartorius muscle (Latin, "of the tailor" so named because it both flexes the knee and rotates the leg outward so that the ankle rests on the knee of the other leg, a postion favored by tailors while sewing clothes)
5 Pectineus muscle
6 Rectus femoris muscle
7 Vastus medialis muscle
8 Vastus lateralis muscle

9 Vastus intermedius muscle; note that the vastus intermedius is covered by the other three muscles (6,7,8) of the quadriceps femoris.
10 Inguinal ligament
11 Tensor fascia lata muscle (supplied by superior gluteal nerve)
12 Adductor longus muscle (supplied by obturator nerve)
13 Gracilis muscle (supplied by obturator nerve)

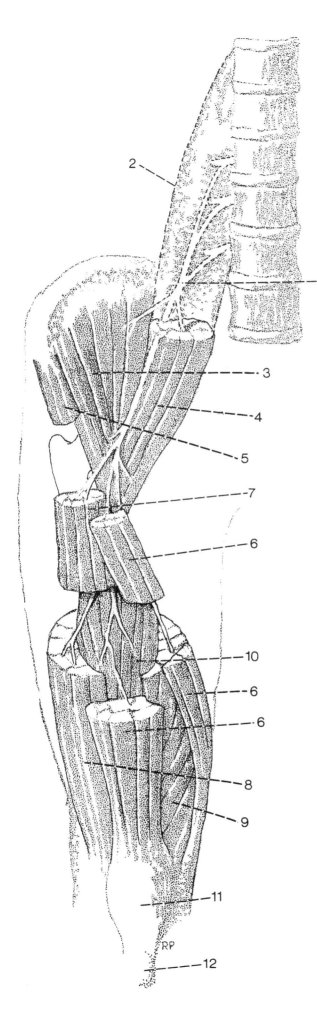

18
Motor distribution of the femoral nerve, II

Color and label

1 Femoral nerve formed by the fibers from lumbar nerves L2, L3, L4
2 Outline of psoas major muscle; notice that the femoral nerve and other nerves of the lumbar plexus arise deep within the substance of the psoas major.
3 Iliacus muscle; it inserts by a tendon in common with the psoas major on the lesser trochanter, thus forming the iliopsoas muscle, which flexes the hip.
4 Psoas major muscle
5 Sartorius muscle; origin on the anterior superior iliac spine (cut)
6 Sartorius muscle (a portion); Sartorius means "tailor's" in Latin, in reference to the sartorius' action in flexing both the hip joint and the knee joint and externally rotating the leg, a position used by tailors when sewing.
7 Rectus femoris muscle (cut)
8 Vastus lateralis muscle (cut)
9 Vastus medialis muscle (cut)
10 Vastus intermedius muscle (cut); the three vastus muscles and the rectus femoris form the quadriceps femoris, which means "four-headed muscle of the thigh".
11 Patella; (knee cap) notice that the patella lies within the tendon of the quadriceps femoris; it is the largest sesamoid bone in the body; the actual insertion of the quadriceps is on the tibial tuberosity by means of the patellar ligament.
12 Tibial tuberosity

19 Deep dissection of right thigh I

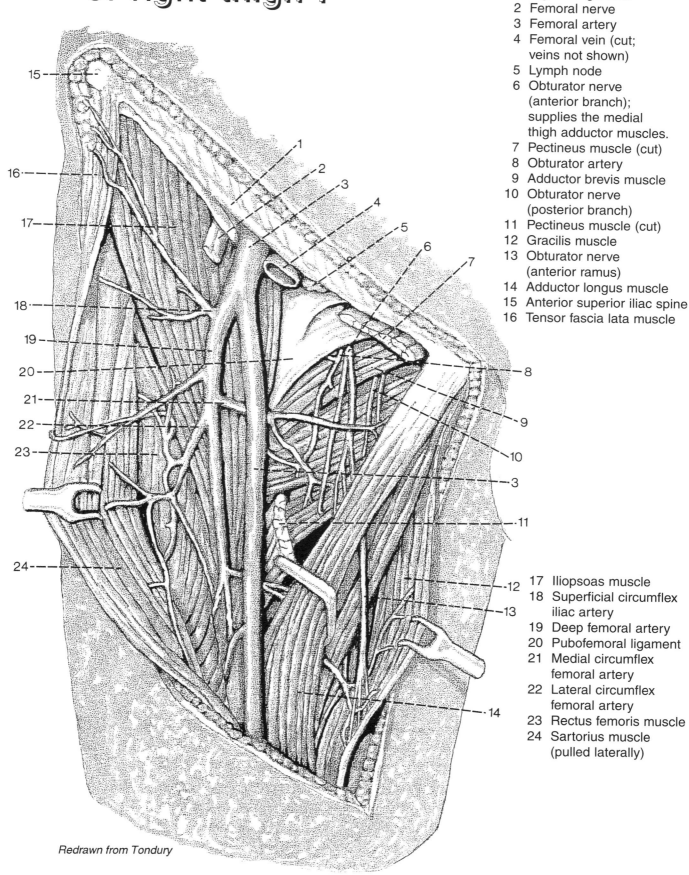

Color and label

1 Inguinal ligament
2 Femoral nerve
3 Femoral artery
4 Femoral vein (cut; veins not shown)
5 Lymph node
6 Obturator nerve (anterior branch); supplies the medial thigh adductor muscles.
7 Pectineus muscle (cut)
8 Obturator artery
9 Adductor brevis muscle
10 Obturator nerve (posterior branch)
11 Pectineus muscle (cut)
12 Gracilis muscle
13 Obturator nerve (anterior ramus)
14 Adductor longus muscle
15 Anterior superior iliac spine
16 Tensor fascia lata muscle

17 Iliopsoas muscle
18 Superficial circumflex iliac artery
19 Deep femoral artery
20 Pubofemoral ligament
21 Medial circumflex femoral artery
22 Lateral circumflex femoral artery
23 Rectus femoris muscle
24 Sartorius muscle (pulled laterally)

Slightly rotated outward

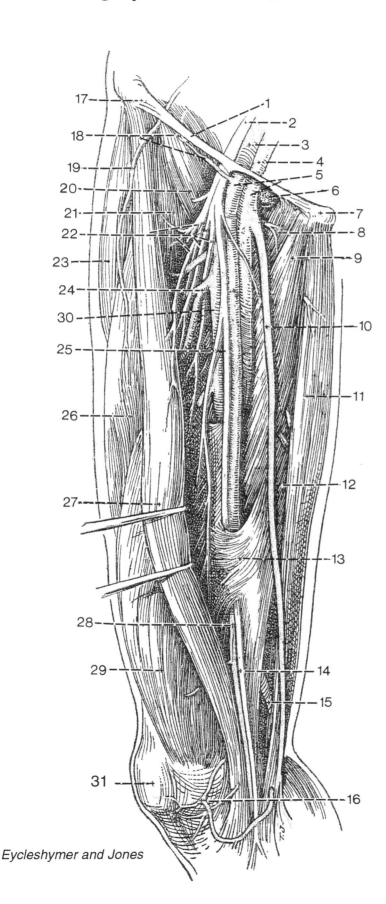

Eycleshymer and Jones

Color and label

1 Inguinal ligament
2 Femoral nerve
3 External iliac artery
4 External iliac vein
5 Femoral artery and vein; note that the **external iliac** artery and vein become the **femoral** artery and vein below the inguinal ligament.
6 Lymph gland
7 Pubic tubercle
8 Pectineus muscle
9 Adductor longus muscle
10 Great saphenous vein (Gk. *saphenes*, visible or clear)
11 Gracilis muscle (L. slender)
12 Adductor magnus muscle
13 Anterior wall of adductor canal (old name, Hunter's canal); a tunnel under the aponeurosis of the adductor magnus transmitting the the femoral vessels, deep lymphatics, and the saphenous nerve.
14 Saphenous nerve
15 Popliteal artery; a continuation of the femoral artery extending from the opening in the adductor magnus, across the floor of the popliteal fossa, to the lower border of the popliteus muscle where it ends by dividing into the anterior and posterior tibial arteries.
16 Medial inferior genicular artery
17 Anterior superior iliac spine
18 Superficial circumflex iliac artery (off femoral artery)
19 Lateral femoral cutaneous nerve
20 Iliopsoas muscle
21 Rectus femoris muscle
22 Motor branches of femoral nerve to muscles
23 Tensor fascia lata muscle; inserts on iliotibial tract
24 Lateral femoral circumflex artery (off deep femoral)
25 Saphenous nerve
26 Rectus femoris muscle
27 Sartorius muscle
28 Medial superior genicular artery
29 Vastus medialis muscle
30 Deep femoral artery
31 Patella

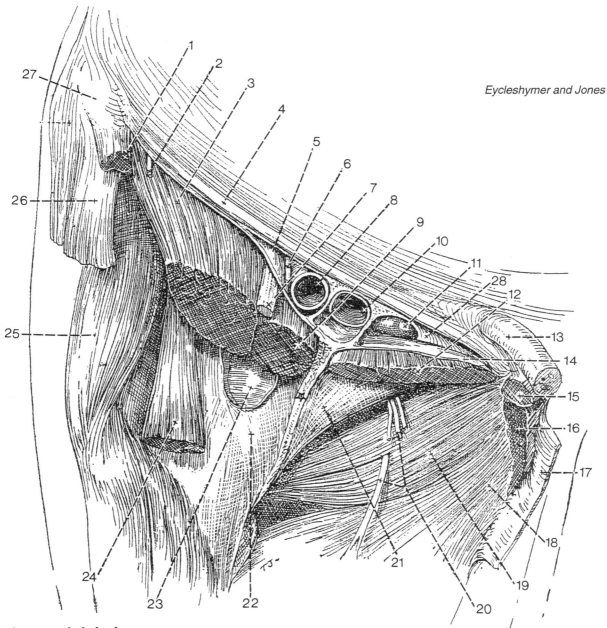

Eycleshymer and Jones

Color and label

1 Sartorius muscle (cut near origin on anterior superior iliac spine)
2 Lateral femoral cutaneous nerve
3 Iliacus muscle
4 Inguinal ligament (old name, Poupart's ligament)
5 Iliopectineal arch; a septum between the inguinal ligament and the iliopectinal eminence of the hip bone that divides the space beneath the inguinal ligament into the lateral muscular lacuna (space) and the medial vascular lacuna.
  Also iliopectineal septum.

6 Femoral branch of genitofemoral nerve
7 Femoral nerve
8 Femoral artery
9 Psoas major muscle
10 Femoral vein
11 Lymph gland
12 Pectineus muscle (cut near its origin on the pecten of the pubic bone)
13 Spermatic cord
14 Pectineal fascia
15 Adductor longus muscle (cut near origin)
16 Adductor brevis (cut near origin)
17 Gracilis muscle (origin, cut)
18 Adductor magnus muscle
19 Obturator externus muscle

20 Obturator nerve; anterior branches (above) posterior branches (below)
21 Pubofemoral ligament
22 Articular capsule of hip joint (also coxal joint, iliofemoral joint, acetabulofemoral joint)
23 Iliopectineal bursa
24 Rectus femoris muscle (cut)
25 Gluteus medius muscle
26 Tensor fascia lata
27 Anterior superior iliac spine
28 Lacunar ligament

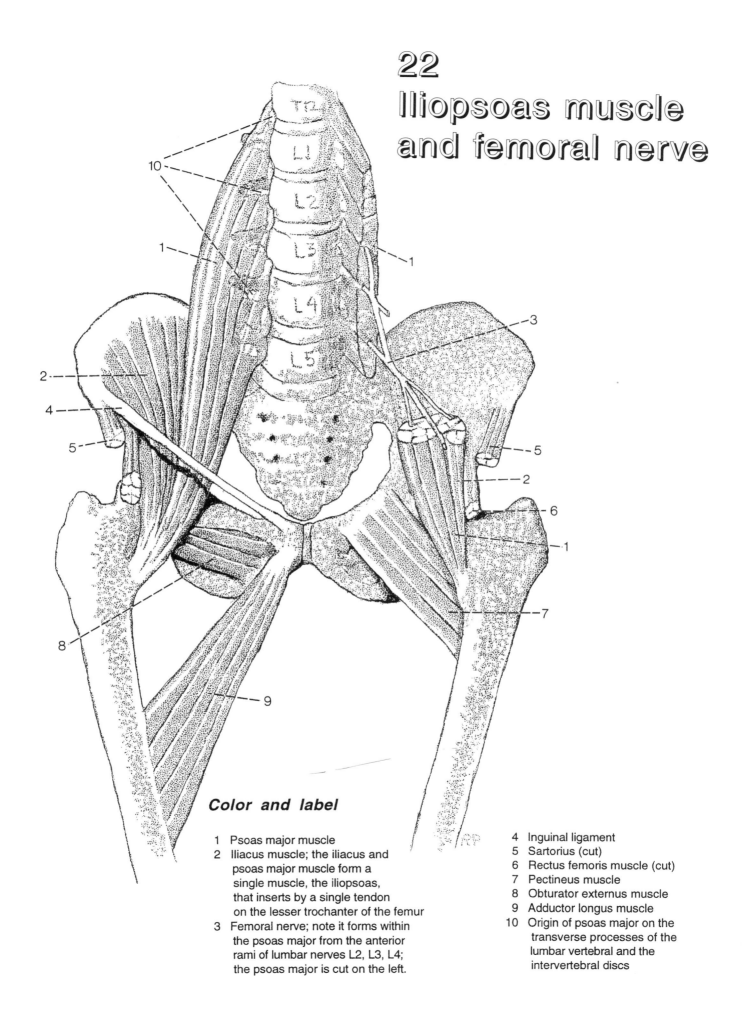

Color and label

1 Psoas major muscle
2 Iliacus muscle; the iliacus and
   psoas major muscle form a
   single muscle, the iliopsoas,
   that inserts by a single tendon
   on the lesser trochanter of the femur
3 Femoral nerve; note it forms within
   the psoas major from the anterior
   rami of lumbar nerves L2, L3, L4;
   the psoas major is cut on the left.

4 Inguinal ligament
5 Sartorius (cut)
6 Rectus femoris muscle (cut)
7 Pectineus muscle
8 Obturator externus muscle
9 Adductor longus muscle
10 Origin of psoas major on the
   transverse processes of the
   lumbar vertebral and the
   intervertebral discs

23 Medial thigh muscles and obturator nerve

Color and label

1 Obturator nerve; note that the obturator nerve, like the femoral nerve, is formed by fibers from the anterior rami of lumbar nerves L2, L3, L4.

2 Anterior branch of obturator nerve; note that this branch passes deep to the pectineus and adductor longus, and in front of the obturator externus which it often penetrates, and the adductor brevis; it supplies the adductor brevis, adductor longus, and gracilis muscles.

3 Pectineus muscle (cut on left side)

4 Obturator externus muscle

5 Adductor brevis and its insertion on the **posterior** femur; note that it lies deep to, and is largely covered by, the pectineus and the adductor longus muscles.

6 Adductor longus and its insertion on the **posterior** femur (cut on left side)

7 Adductor magnus muscle (oblique part); the adductor magnus is really a double muscle; this part is innerveted by the posterior branch of the obturator nerve.

8 Adductor magnus muscle (vertical part); this part is innerveted by the tibial division of the sciatic nerve; note this part's insertion on the adductor tubercle.

9 Gracilis muscle (cut on left)

10 Tendineus hiatus; opening in the tendon of the adductor magnus for the passage of the femoral vessels from the femoral canal to the popliteal fossa

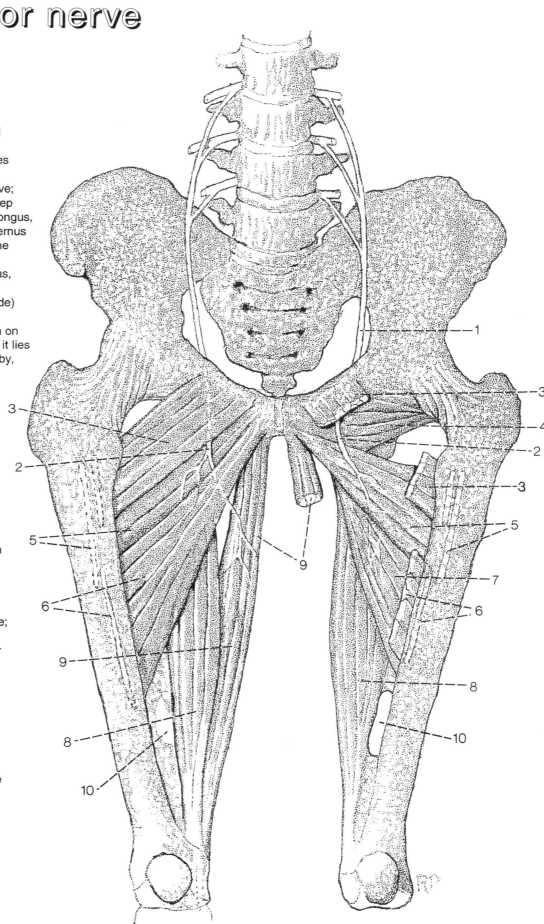

24 Adductor magnus and obturator nerve

Color and label

1 Obturator nerve; it arises within the psoas major muscle (removed) from the anterior rami of lumbar nerves L2, L3, L4; it divides into an anterior branch and posterior branch which both pass through the obturator foramen.
2 Anterior branch of obturator nerve (cut)
3 Posterior branch of obturator nerve; note its passing through the obturator externus muscle which it also supplies.
4 Adductor magnus muscle (anterior horizontal part); this part of the adductor magnus is sometimes considered a separate muscle in which case it is called the adductor minimus.
5 Adductor magnus muscle (anterior oblique part); the anterior horizontal and oblique parts of the adductor magnus are supplied by the posterior branch of the obturator nerve.
6 Adductor magnus (posterior vertical part); this part arises from the ischial tuberosity, descends vertically, forms a tendon that inserts on the adductor tubercle of the femur; the vertical part is innervated by the tibial portion of the sciatic nerve.

7 Femoral nerve and artery (a section of each) passing through the tendineus hiatus (also adductor hiatus)
8 Fibrous expansion of adductor magnus tendon
9 Pectineus muscle (cut); usually supplied by the femoral nerve, sometimes by the obturator nerve or accessory obturator nerve.
10 Obturator externus muscle; shown passing behind the femur and inserting into its trochanter fossa
11 Outline of the anterior part of adductor magnus; note its insertion on the posterior femur
12 Accessory obturator nerve; present 10% of the time; notice it passes over the pubis and not through the obturator foramen.
13 Obturator* foramen
14 Insertion of anterior part of obturator magnus on gluteal ridge and linea aspera of the femur
15 Insertion of iliopsoas tendon on lesser trochanter
16 Origin of pectineus

*From the Latin, *obturare*, to obstruct or stop up

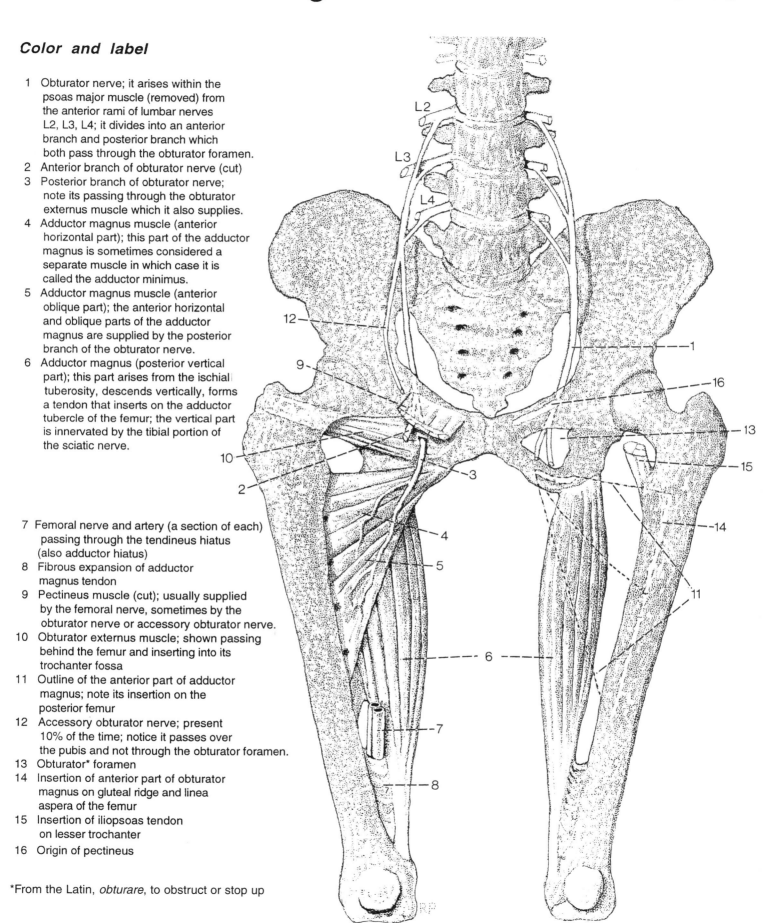

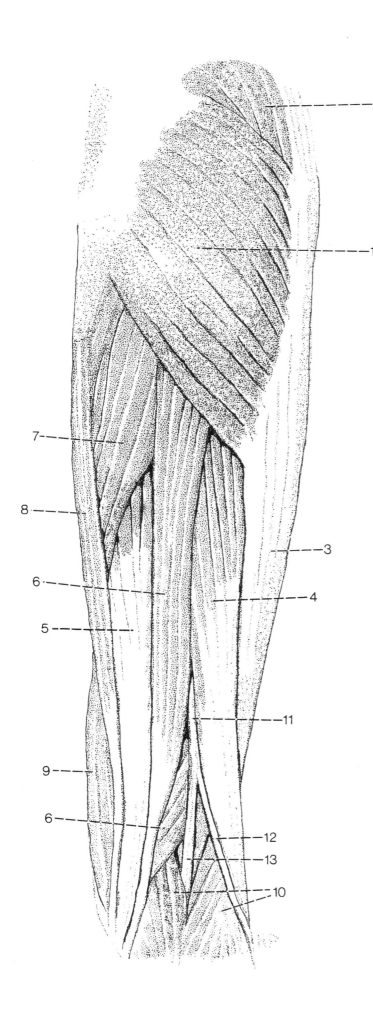

25
Muscles of buttock and posterior thigh

RIGHT THIGH

Color and label

1 Gluteus maximus
2 Gluteus medius
3 Iliotibial tract; note that the gluteus maximus inserts mainly on the iliotibial tract
4 Biceps femoris (the lateral hamstring muscle)
5 Semitendinosus (medial hamstring muscle)
6 Semimembranosus
7 Adductor magnus (posterior vertical part)
8 Gracilis
9 Sartorius
10 Medial and lateral heads of gastrocnemius
11 Sciatic nerve; its division into the tibial and common peroneal (fibular) nerves may occur higher in the thigh.
12 Common peroneal (fibular) nerve
13 Tibial nerve

26 Gluteus maximus and iliotibial tract

Right leg, posterior view

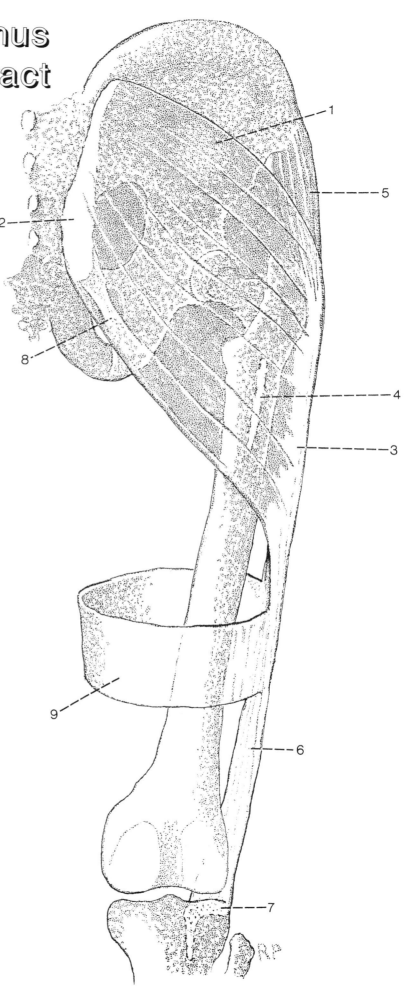

Color and label

1 Gluteus maximus; (largest and most superficial muscle in the gluteal region).

2 Origin of gluteus maximus; from ilium and lower part of sacrum; it also arises from the coccyx, aponeurosis of erector spinae, and sacrotuberous ligament (8).

3 Insertion of gluteus maximus on iliotibial tract; besides being a powerful extensor of the thigh at the hip and rotator of the thigh, the gluteus maximus, acting by way of its insertion on the iliotibial tract, braces the fully extended knee (as in standing).

4 Insertion of lower deeper fibers of gluteus maximus on gluteal tuberosity of femur.

5 Tensor fascia lata muscle

6 Iliotibial tract (lateral thickened portion of fascia lata)

7 Insertion of iliotibial tract on anterior surface of lateral condyle of tibia

8 Sacrotuberous ligament

9 Small section of fascia lata (deep fascia of the thigh)

27 Posterior gluteal and thigh muscles

Right leg

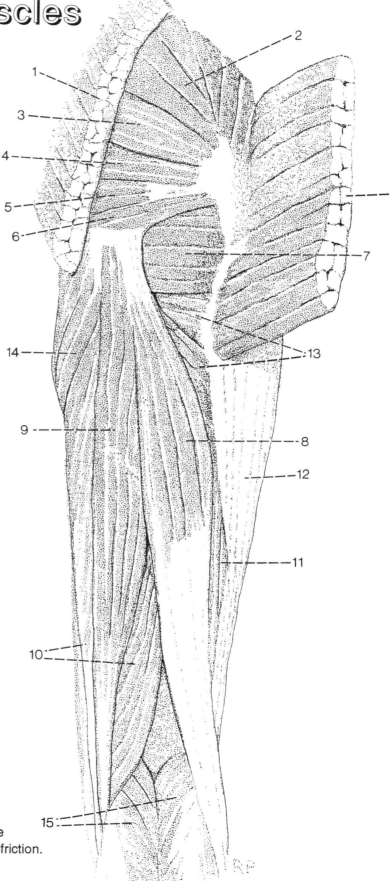

Color and label

1 Gluteus maximus
2 Gluteus medius;
   intermuscular
   gluteal bursae*
   have been removed
3 Piriformis
4 Superior gemellus
5 Obturator internus
6 Inferior gemellus
7 Quadratus femoris
8 Biceps femoris
   (long head)
9 Semitendinosus
10 Semimembranosus
11 Biceps femoris
   (short head)
12 Iliotibial tract
13 Adductor magnus
   (oblique part)
14 Adductor magnus
   (vertical part)
15 Gastrocnemius medial
   and lateral heads

*Bursa (L. a bag or purse):
a closed sac or pouch lined with synovial membrane
containing synovial fluid formed in areas subject to friction.

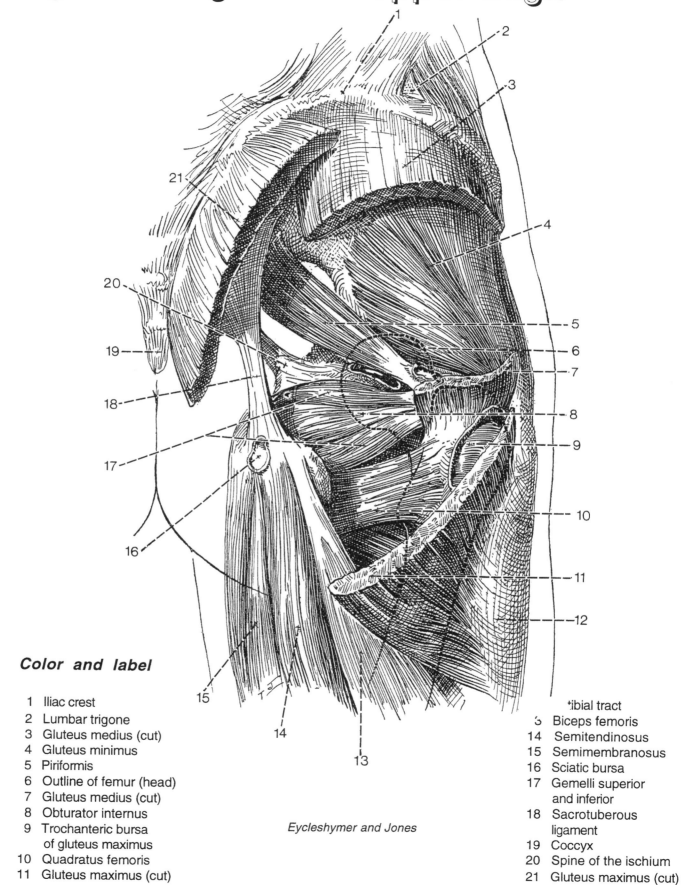

Eycleshymer and Jones

Color and label

1 Iliac crest
2 Lumbar trigone
3 Gluteus medius (cut)
4 Gluteus minimus
5 Piriformis
6 Outline of femur (head)
7 Gluteus medius (cut)
8 Obturator internus
9 Trochanteric bursa
   of gluteus maximus
10 Quadratus femoris
11 Gluteus maximus (cut)

Tibial tract
12 Biceps femoris
14 Semitendinosus
15 Semimembranosus
16 Sciatic bursa
17 Gemelli superior
    and inferior
18 Sacrotuberous
    ligament
19 Coccyx
20 Spine of the ischium
21 Gluteus maximus (cut)

29 Deep gluteal region

Right leg posterior aspect

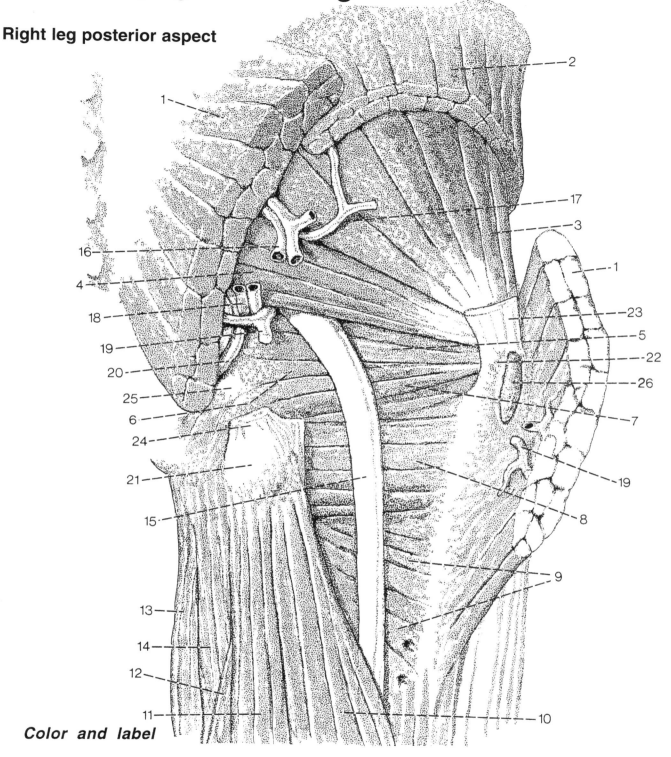

Color and label

1	Gluteus maximus muscle (cut)
2	Gluteus medius muscle (cut)
3	Gluteus minimus muscle (cut)
4	Piriformis muscle
5	Superior gemellus muscle
6	Obturator internus muscle
7	Inferior gemellus muscle
8	Quadratus femoris muscle
9	Adductor magnus (horizontal and oblique parts)
10	Biceps femoris muscle
11	Semitendinosus muscle
12	Semimembranosus muscle
13	Gracilis muscle
14	Adductor magnus muscle (vertical part)
15	Sciatic nerve
16	Superior gluteal artery and vein
17	Superior gluteal nerve (cut; supplies gluteus medius and gluteus minimus)
18	Inferior gluteal artery and vein
19	Inferior gluteal nerve (supplies gluteus maximus)
20	Internal pudendal artery and vein (travel with pudendal nerve; nerve not shown)
21	Ischial tuberosity
22	Greater trochanter of femur
23	Tendon of gluteus medius
24	Sacrotuberous ligament (cut)
25	Bend (genu) in obturator internus muscle on lesser sciatic notch
26	Trochanteric bursa (beneath gluteus maximus)

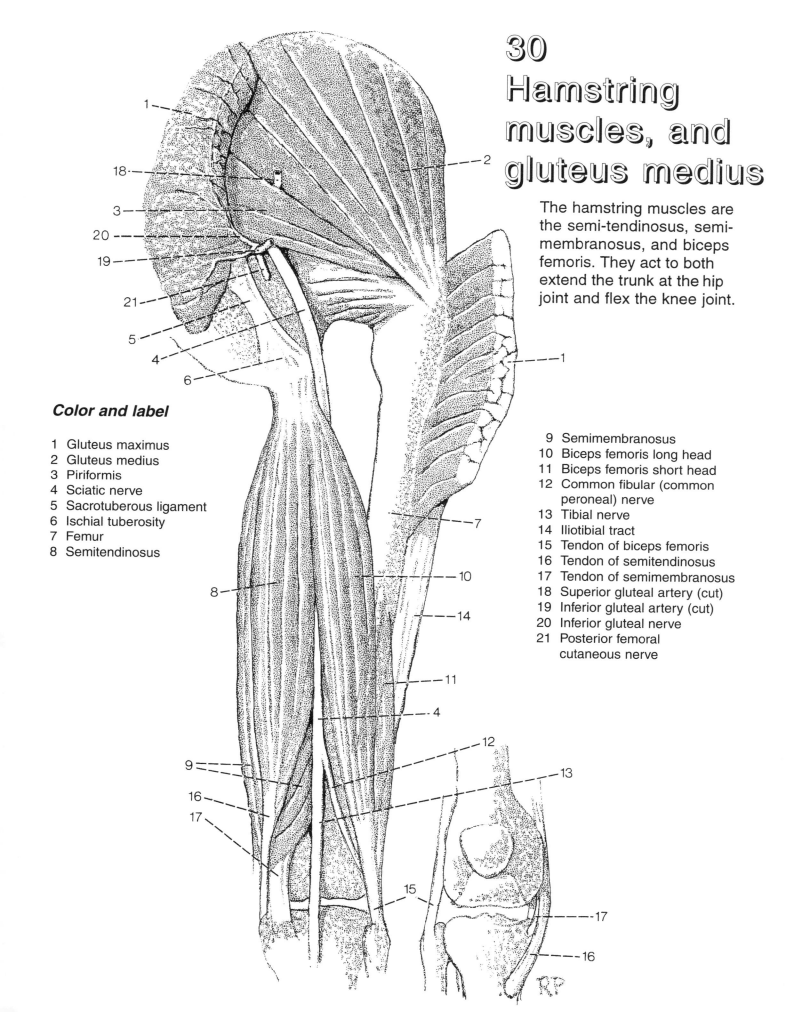

The hamstring muscles are the semi-tendinosus, semi-membranosus, and biceps femoris. They act to both extend the trunk at the hip joint and flex the knee joint.

Color and label

1 Gluteus maximus
2 Gluteus medius
3 Piriformis
4 Sciatic nerve
5 Sacrotuberous ligament
6 Ischial tuberosity
7 Femur
8 Semitendinosus

9   Semimembranosus
10 Biceps femoris long head
11 Biceps femoris short head
12 Common fibular (common peroneal) nerve
13 Tibial nerve
14 Iliotibial tract
15 Tendon of biceps femoris
16 Tendon of semitendinosus
17 Tendon of semimembranosus
18 Superior gluteal artery (cut)
19 Inferior gluteal artery (cut)
20 Inferior gluteal nerve
21 Posterior femoral cutaneous nerve

31 Gluteus minimus, semimembranosus, and sciatic nerve

Posterior aspect

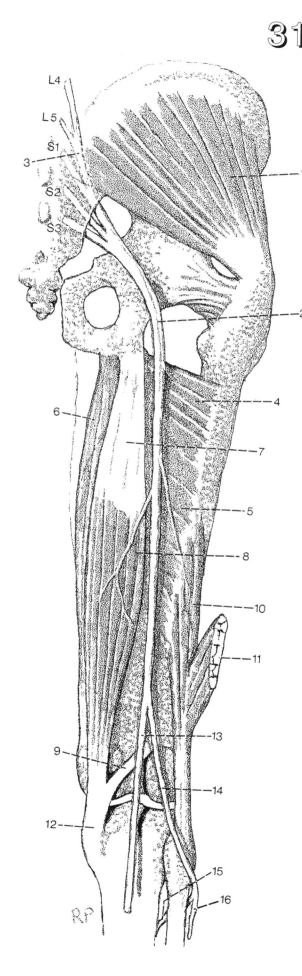

Color and label

1 Gluteus minimus muscle; it works in concert with the gluteus medius to stabilize the pelvis when the opposite leg is off the ground, thereby maintaining the trunk upright.
2 Sciatic nerve (viewed through a transparent sacrum; note how it arises from spinal nerves L4, L5, S1,S2, S3)
3 Lumbosacral trunk; conveys fibers from lumbar nerves L4 and L5 to the sciatic nerve.
4 Adductor magnus muscle (horizontal part)
5 Adductor magnus muscle (oblique part)
6 Adductor magnus muscle (vertical part)
7 Flat tendon of semimembranosus muscle; this flat tendon gives this muscle its name.
8 Semimembranosus muscle (muscular part)
9 Oblique popliteal ligament
10 Short head of biceps femoris muscle; innervated by common peroneal nerve (common fibular nerve)
11 Long head of biceps femoris muscle (cut)
12 Semimembranosus insertion onto the back of the medial condyle of the tibia; also onto the the lateral femoral condyle by the oblique popliteal ligament
13 Tibial nerve
14 Common peroneal nerve (common fibular nerve)
15 Deep peroneal nerve (deep fibular nerve)
16 Superficial peroneal nerve (superficial fibular nerve)

32 Deep dissection of the right thigh

Posterior aspect

Color and label

1 Crest of the ilium
2 Gluteus medius muscle (cut)
3 Superior gluteal artery
  (vein not shown)
4 Superior gluteal nerve
5 Piriformis muscle
6 Inferior gluteal nerve
7 Inferior gluteal artery
8 Gluteus medius muscle (cut);
  inserting on the greater trochanter
9 Posterior femoral cutaneus nerve
10 Sciatic nerve; largest nerve
  in the body, consisting of a medial
  tibial nerve and a lateral common
  fibular (peroneal) nerve
11 Superior gemellus muscle
12 Obturator internus muscle
13 Inferior gemellus muscle
14 Greater trochanter of femur
15 Quadratus femoris muscle
16 Gluteus maximus (cut); inserting
  on iliotibial tract
17 Adductor magnus muscle (horizontal part)
18 First perforating branch of deep
  femoral artery
19 Inferior clunial nerve
20 Second perforating branch of
  deep femoral nerve
21 Adductor magnus muscle (oblique part)
22 Branch of common fibular
  (peroneal) nerve to short head
  of the biceps femoris muscle
23 Third perforating artery of the deep
  femoral artery
24 Iliotibial tract
25 Biceps femoris muscle (long head, cut)
26 Popliteal artery (continuation of
  femoral artery)
27 Popliteal vein (continuation of
  femoral vein)
28 Tibial nerve
29 Adductor magnus muscle
30 Gracilis muscle
31 Short head of biceps femoris muscle
32 Common fibular (peroneal) nerve

Eycleshymer and Jones with modification

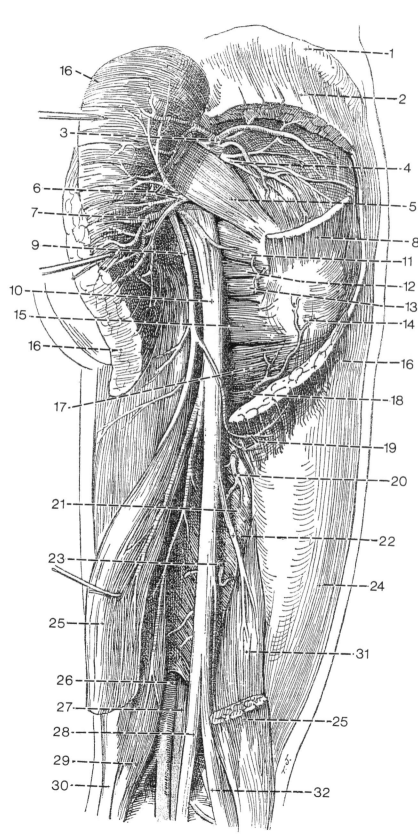

33 Cross section of right thigh

Middle of right thigh

Color and label

1 Femur
2 Sciatic nerve
3 Fascia lata (deep fascia of thigh)
4 Iliotibial tract (thickened fascia lata)
5 Great saphenous vein
6 Femoral artery, vein, and saphenous nerve
   in adductor canal
7 Deep femoral artery and vein
8 Perforating vessels
9 Posterior femoral cutaneous nerve
10 Lateral femoral cutaneous nerve
11 Anterior branch of obturator nerve
12 Rectus femoris
13 Vastus lateralis
14 Vastus medialis
15 Vastus intermedius
16 Gracilis
17 Sartorius
18 Biceps femoris, long head
19 Semitendinosus
20 Semimembranosus
21 Adductor magnus
22 Adductor longus

Posterior Compartment
tibial nerve

Anterior Compartment
femoral nerve

Medial Compartment
obturator nerve

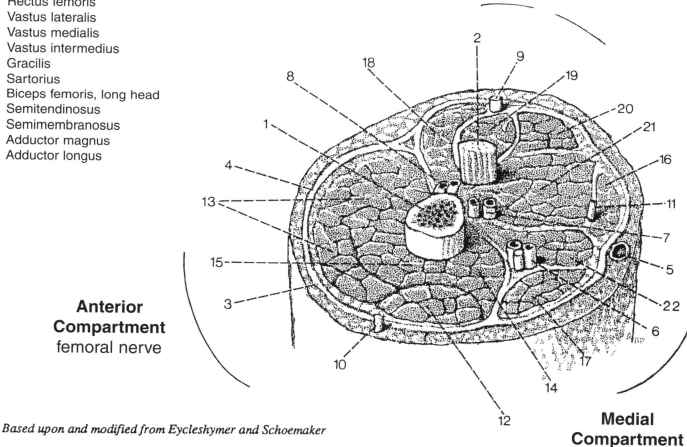

Based upon and modified from Eycleshymer and Schoemaker

Notice that the deep fascia of the thigh, which is called the fascia lata, sends septa internally that divide the thigh into three compartments, a medial, an anterior, and a posterior compartment. The femoral nerve innervates the muscles of the anterior compartment, the obturator nerve supplies the muscles of the medial compartment, and the tibial portion of the sciatic nerve supplies the muscles of the posterior compartment.

34 Deep structures of the leg and popliteal fossa

Gastrocnemius and soleus removed showing course of popliteal artery and tibial nerve

Color and label

1 Sciatic nerve
2 Biceps femoris
3 Common fibular nerve
4 Tibial nerve
5 Gastrocnemius
   lateral head (cut)
6 Sural artery and nerve
7 Lateral superior
   genicular artery
8 Semimembranosus
9 Popliteal artery
   (vein not shown)
10 Gracilis muscle
11 Gastrocnemius
    medial head (cut)
12 Artery and nerve to
    gastrocnemius
13 Medial superior
    genicular artery
14 Popliteus muscle
15 Soleus muscle (cut)
16 Fibular (peroneal) artery
17 Flexor hallucis
    longus muscle
18 Fibular (peroneus)
    longus muscle
19 Fibular (peroneus)
    brevis muscle
20 Sural nerve
21 Lateral malleolar artery
22 Flexor digitorum longus muscle
23 Tibialis posterior muscle
24 Posterior tibial artery
25 Calcaneal (Achilles) tendon

Eycleshymer and Jones

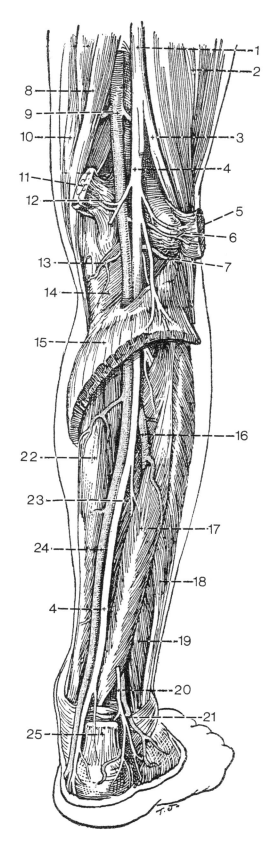

Posterior aspect

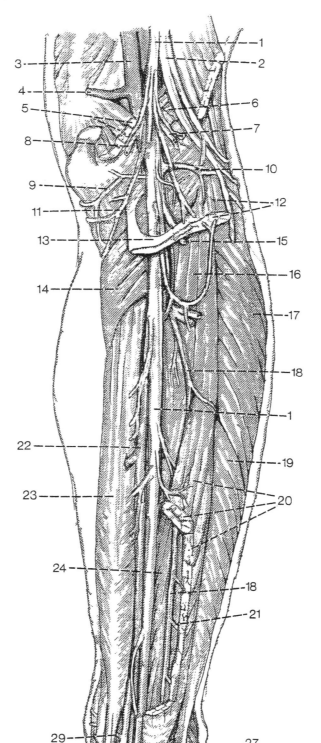

Color and label

1 Tibial nerve
2 Common fibular (peroneal) nerve
3 Popliteal artery
4 Medial superior genicular artery
5 Gastrocnemius muscle
   (medial head; cut)
6 Gastrocnemius (lateral head; cut)
7 Lateral sural nerve and artery
8 Medial sural artery and nerve
9 Medial inferior genicular artery
10 Lateral inferior genicular artery
11 Medial sural cutaneous nerve
12 Soleus muscle (cut)
13 Tendinous arch (part of soleus)
14 Popliteus muscle
15 Anterior tibial artery
16 Tibialis posterior muscle
17 Peroneus (fibularis) longus
   muscle

18 Peroneal (fibular) artery
19 Peroneus (fibularis) brevis
   muscle
20 Flexor hallucis longus
   muscle; partially dissected
   to reveal the underlying
   peroneal artery
21 Perforating branch of the
   peroneal artery
22 Posterior tibial artery
23 Flexor digitorum longus muscle
24 Tibialis posterior
25 Calcaneal (Achilles) tendon
26 Medial calcaneal artery
27 Lateral malleolar artery
28 Lateral calcaneal artery
29 Medial malleolar artery

*In anatomy the term **leg** designates
just that portion of the lower limb
below the knee and above the foot.
The **thigh** designates the upper
portion extending from the hip
to the knee.

*Redrawn from Clemente, Gray's Anatomy
30th American Ed. Lea & Febiger 1985
Philadelphia*

Right leg

Color and label

1 Fascia lata (deep fascia of thigh)
2 Biceps femoris (long head)
3 Common fibular (peroneal) nerve
4 Tibial nerve
5 Popliteal artery
6 Popliteal vein
7 Gastrocnemius muscle (lateral head)
8 Plantaris muscle
9 Soleus muscle (cut)
10 Common fibular (peroneal) nerve
11 Anterior tibial artery
12 Anterior tibial vein
13 Fibula
14 Soleus muscle
15 Gastrocnemius muscle
16 Tendon of plantaris muscle
17 Tibial nerve
18 Popliteus muscle
19 Tendon of semimembranous muscle
20 Gastrocnemius muscle (medial head)
21 Oblique popliteal ligament
22 Adductor magnus muscle
23 Semitendinosus muscle
24 Semimembranosus muscle

Redrawn from Tondury

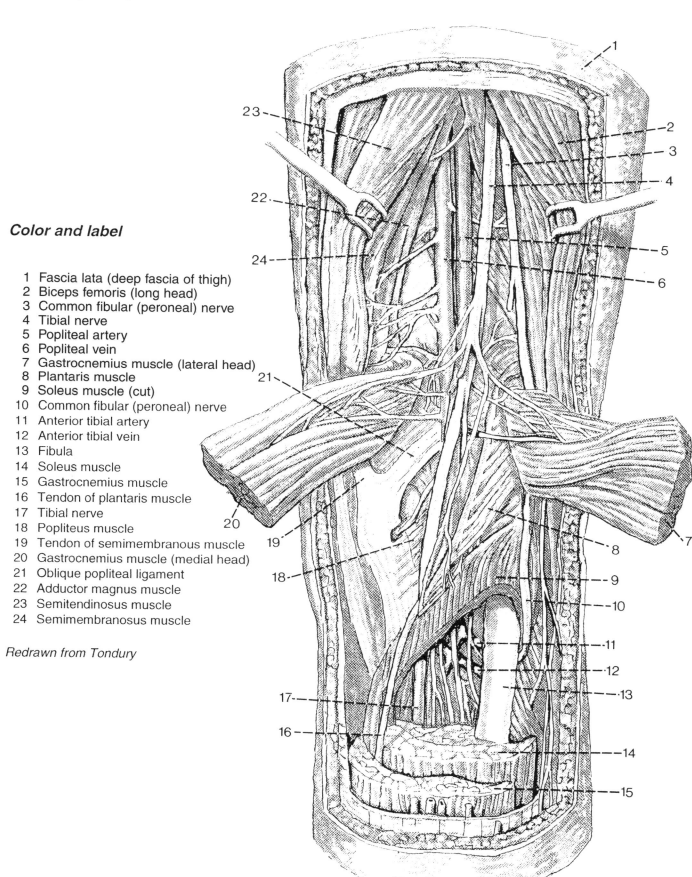

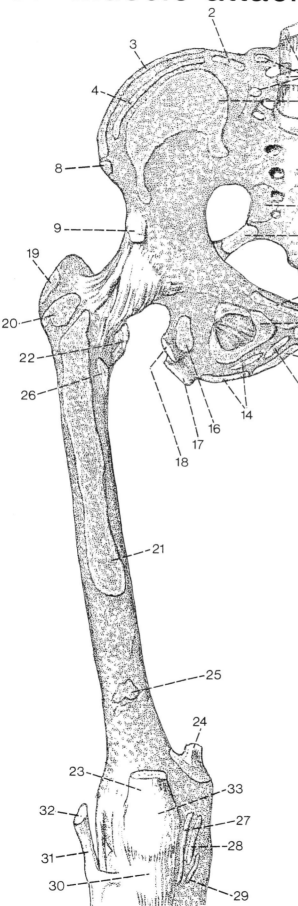

**Color the origins (O) RED
and the insertions (I) BLUE**

1 Psoas major (O)
2 Quadratus lumborum (O)
3 Internal abdominal oblique (O)
4 Transversus abdominis (O)
5 Iliacus (O)
6 Piriformis (O)
7 Coccygeus (O) on sacrospinous ligament
8 Sartorius (O)
9 Rectus femoris (O) straight head
10 Pectineus (O)
11 Adductor longus (O)
12 Adductor brevis (O)
13 Gracilis (O)
14 Adductor magnus (O)
15 Obturator externus (O)
16 Quadratus femoris (O)
17 Semimembranosus (O)
18 Biceps femoris (O)
19 Gluteus minimus (I)
20 Vastus lateralis (O)
21 Vastus intermedius (O)
22 Iliopsoas (I)
23 Quadriceps femoris (I)
24 Adductor magnus (I)
25 Articularis genu (O)
26 Vastus medialis (O)
27 Sartorius (I)
28 Gracilis (I)
29 Semitendinosus (I)
30 Patellar ligament
31 Fibular collateral ligament
32 Biceps femoris (I)
33 Patella

After Clemente.

Color the origins (O) RED and the insertions (I) BLUE

1 External abdominal oblique (I)
2 Gluteus medius (O)
3 Gluteus minimus (O)
4 Gluteus maximus (O) arising on posterior sacroiliac ligament and sacrotuberous ligament
5 Tensor fascia lata (O)
6 Piriformis (O)
7 Rectus femoris oblique head (O)
8 Gemellus superior (O)
9 Gemellus inferior (O)
10 Obturator internus (O)
11 Levator ani (pubococcygeus) (O)
12 Deep transverse perineus (in male) (O)
13 Piriformis (I)
14 Obturator internus with two gemelli (I)
15 Gluteus medius (I)
16 Gluteus minimus (I)
17 Obturator externus (I)
18 Quadratus femoris (I)
19 Iliopsoas (I)
20 Vastus medialis (O)
21 Pectineus (I)
22 Adductor brevis (I)
23 Gluteus maximus
24 Vastus lateralis (O)
25 Vastus intermedius (O)
26 Adductor longus (I)
27 Adductor magnus (I) (anterior oblique part)
28 Biceps femoris short head (O)
29 Plantaris (O)
30 Gastrocnemius (lateral and medial heads) (O)
31 Biceps femoris (I)
32 Semimembranosus (I) *(inserts by three tendons)*
33 Sartorius (I)
34 Gracilis (I)
35 Semitendinosus (I)
36 Semitendinosus (O)
37 Biceps femoris (O)
38 Adductor magnus (I) (posterior vertical part)

After Clemente.

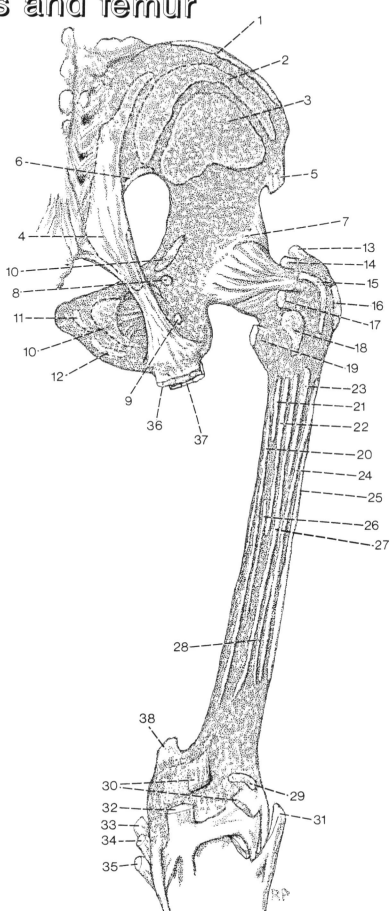

39 Lumbosacral plexus

Right

The shaded nerves are dorsal derivatives of the plexus. These originally innervated dorsal extensor muscles.

Color and label

T12, subcostal nerve (twelfth thoracic nerve, ventral ramus)
L1-L5, ventral rami of lumbar nerves 1-5
S1-S5, ventral rami of sacral nerves 1-5
Co, coccygeal nerve

1 Rami to intertransversarii muscle
2 Rami to quadratus lumborum muscle
3 Iliohypogastric nerve
4 Ilioinguinal nerve
5 Lateral cutaneous branch
6 Genitofemoral nerve
7 Femoral branch of genitofemoral nerve
8 Genital branch of genitofemoral nerve
9 Ramus to psoas minor muscle
10 Ramus to psoas major muscle
11 Femoral nerve
12 Branch to iliacus muscle (of femoral nerve)
13 Anterior cutaneous branch (of femoral nerve)
and branch to sartorius muscle (of femoral nerve)
14 Branch to quadriceps femoris muscle (of femoral nerve)
15 Saphenous nerve (of femoral nerve)
16 Medial femoral cutaneous branch (of femoral nerve)
17 Branch to pectineus muscle (of femoral nerve)
18 Branch to pectineus and psoas major muscles
19 Accessory obturator nerve *(present in about 10% of legs examined)*
20 Obturator nerve
21 Lumbosacral trunk
22 Superior gluteal nerve
23 Rami to piriformis muscle
24 Peroneal nerve (common peroneal nerve)
25 Inferior gluteal nerve
26 Tibial nerve *(the tibial nerve and the common peroneal nerve usually combine to form the largest nerve in the body, the sciatic nerve)*
27 Branch of tibial nerve to adductor magnus (posterior part), semimembranosus, semitendinosus, and long head of biceps femoris muscles
28 Branch to quadratus femoris and gemellus inferior muscles
29 Branch to obturator internus and gemellus superior muscles
30 Posterior femoral cutaneous nerves
31 Inferior cluneal nerve
32 Perineal nerve and dorsal nerve of penis (clitoris)
33 Inferior rectal nerve
34 Branch to levator ani muscle
35 Branch to coccygeus muscle
36 Anococcygeal nerves
37 Lateral femoral cutaneous nerve

After Spalteholz and Spanner (Eisler).

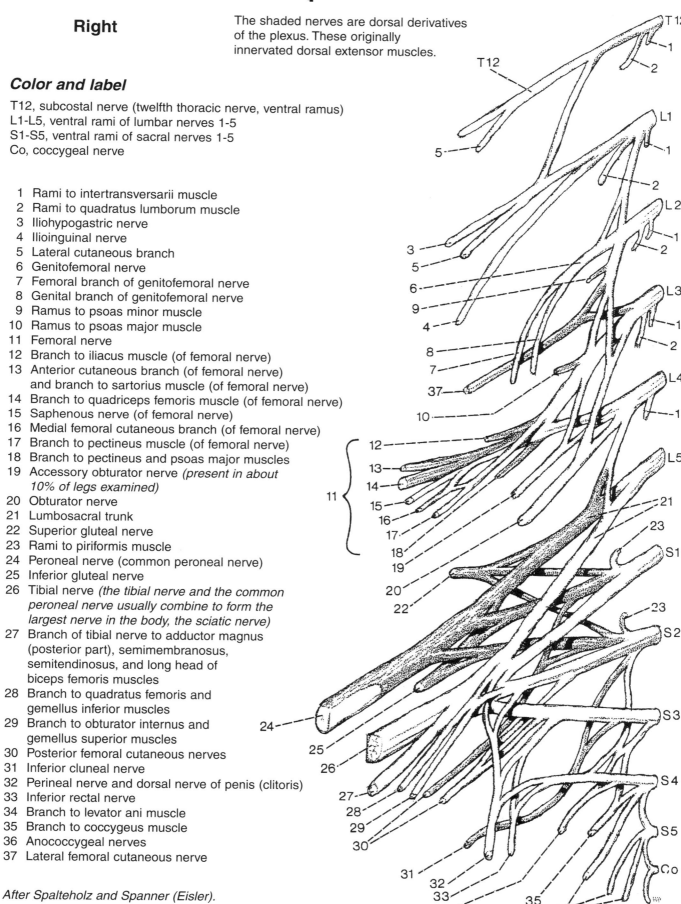

40 Gastrocnemius

Color and label

1 Gastrocnemius (origin of medial head)
2 Gastrocnemius (origin of lateral head)
3 Femur
4 Gastrocnemius
5 Tendo calcaneus (Achilles tendon)
6 Insertion of gastrocnemius and soleus
   (triceps surae) on calcaneus
7 Tibial nerve
8 Common peroneal nerve (common fibular nerve)

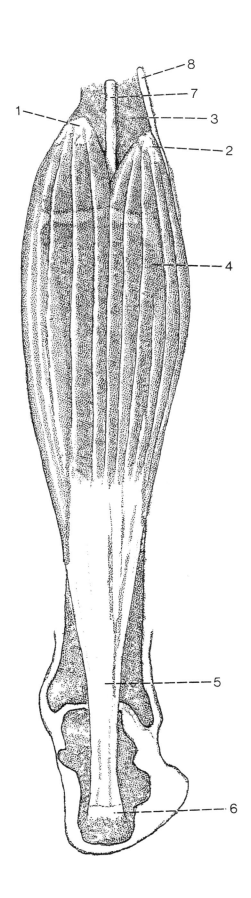

Right leg, posterior view

Color and label

1 Medial head of gastrocnemius *(cut)*
2 Lateral head of gastrocnemius *(cut)*
3 Plantaris *(this muscle is small and almost insignificant in the human)*
4 Tendon of plantaris *(long and thin and easily mistaken for a nerve; it may combine with the tendo calcaneus or insert separately on the tubercle of the calcaneus)*
5 Soleus *(it, along with the two heads of the gastrocnemius, inserts by the tendo calcaneus on the tubercle of the calcaneus; the term triceps surae [Latin for "three heads of the calf"] refers to the two heads of the gastrocnemius and the soleus)*
6 Outline of the gastrocnemius
7 Tibia
8 Fibula
9 Tendo calcaneus
10 Insertion of tendo calcaneus

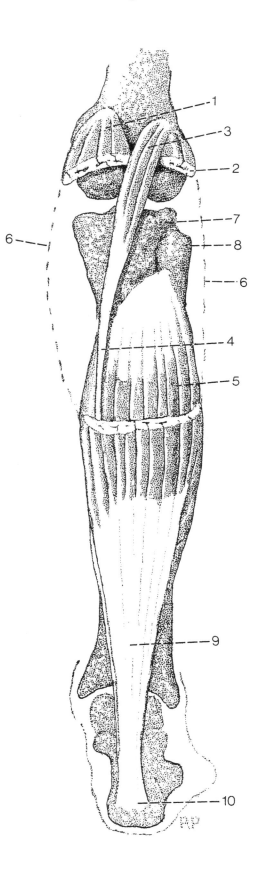

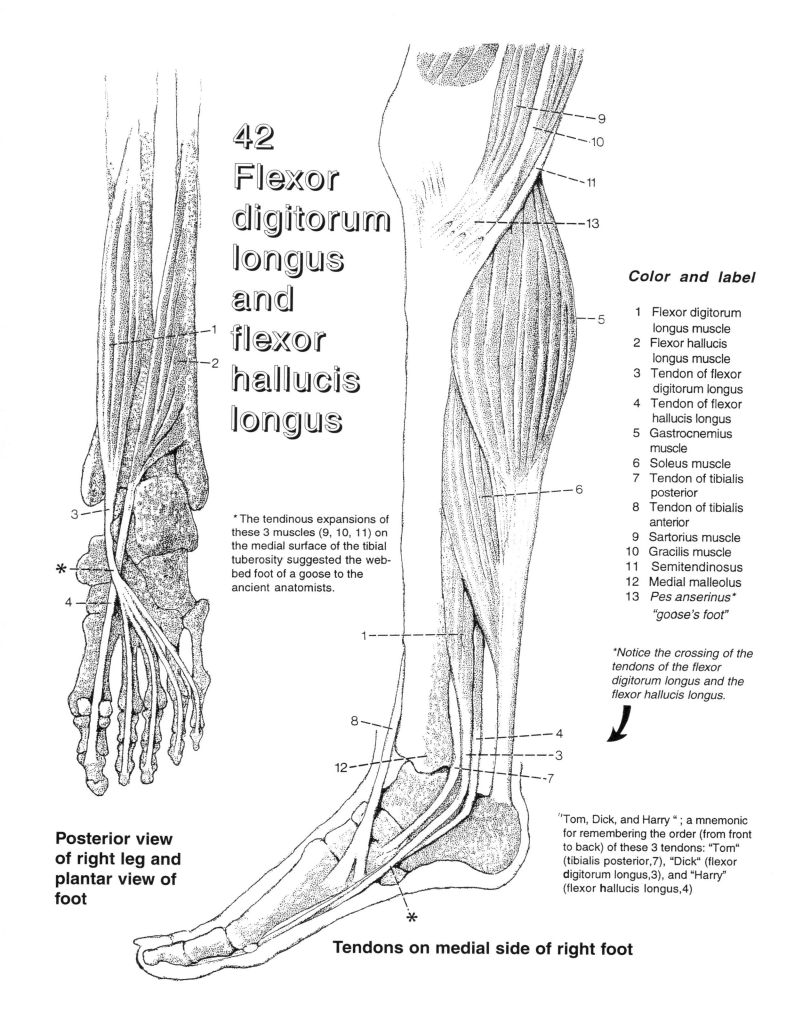

42
Flexor digitorum longus and flexor hallucis longus

* The tendinous expansions of these 3 muscles (9, 10, 11) on the medial surface of the tibial tuberosity suggested the web-bed foot of a goose to the ancient anatomists.

Color and label

1 Flexor digitorum longus muscle
2 Flexor hallucis longus muscle
3 Tendon of flexor digitorum longus
4 Tendon of flexor hallucis longus
5 Gastrocnemius muscle
6 Soleus muscle
7 Tendon of tibialis posterior
8 Tendon of tibialis anterior
9 Sartorius muscle
10 Gracilis muscle
11 Semitendinosus
12 Medial malleolus
13 *Pes anserinus** *"goose's foot"*

*Notice the crossing of the tendons of the flexor digitorum longus and the flexor hallucis longus.

"Tom, Dick, and Harry "; a mnemonic for remembering the order (from front to back) of these 3 tendons: "Tom" (**t**ibialis posterior,7), "Dick" (flexor **d**igitorum longus,3), and "Harry" (flexor **h**allucis longus,4)

Posterior view of right leg and plantar view of foot

Tendons on medial side of right foot

43 Deep muscles in the posterior leg compartment

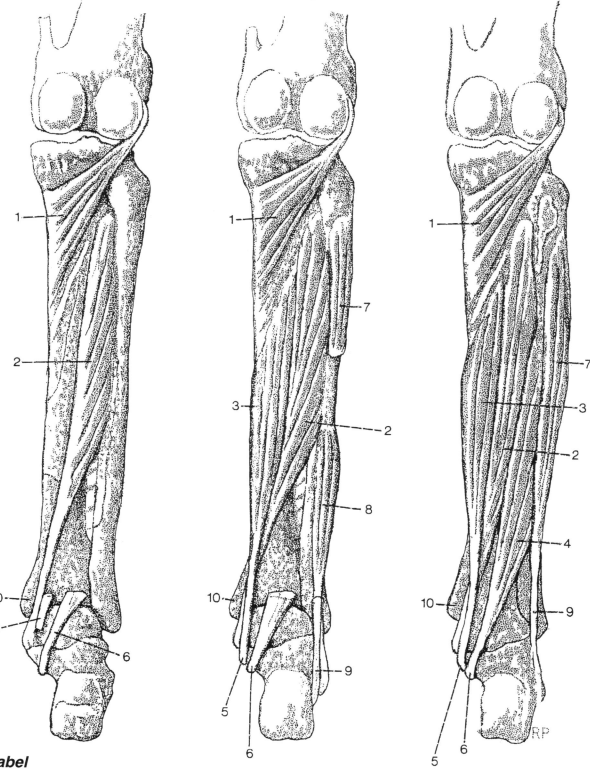

Right leg

Color and label

1 Popliteus
2 Tibialis posterior
3 Flexor digitorum longus
4 Flexor hallucis longus
5 Tendon of flexor digitorum longus

6 Tendon of flexor hallucis longus
7 Peroneus longus (lateral compartment)
8 Peroneus brevis (lateral compartment)
9 Tendon of pereoneus longus
10 Medial malleolus

44 Flexor hallucis longus

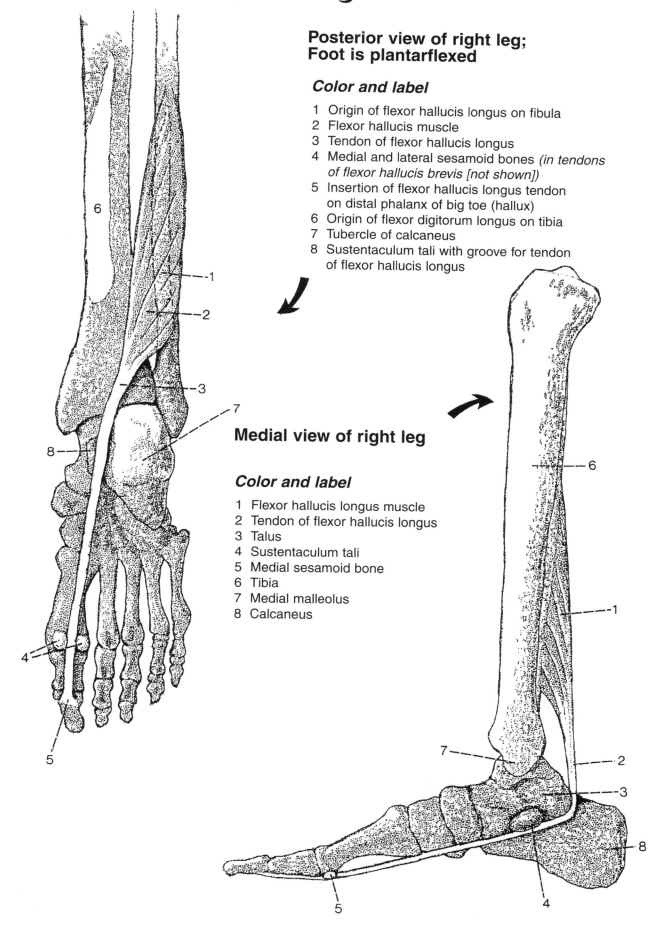

**Posterior view of right leg;
Foot is plantarflexed**

Color and label

1 Origin of flexor hallucis longus on fibula
2 Flexor hallucis muscle
3 Tendon of flexor hallucis longus
4 Medial and lateral sesamoid bones *(in tendons of flexor hallucis brevis [not shown])*
5 Insertion of flexor hallucis longus tendon on distal phalanx of big toe (hallux)
6 Origin of flexor digitorum longus on tibia
7 Tubercle of calcaneus
8 Sustentaculum tali with groove for tendon of flexor hallucis longus

Medial view of right leg

Color and label

1 Flexor hallucis longus muscle
2 Tendon of flexor hallucis longus
3 Talus
4 Sustentaculum tali
5 Medial sesamoid bone
6 Tibia
7 Medial malleolus
8 Calcaneus

45 Muscles of lateral leg

Lateral aspect of right leg

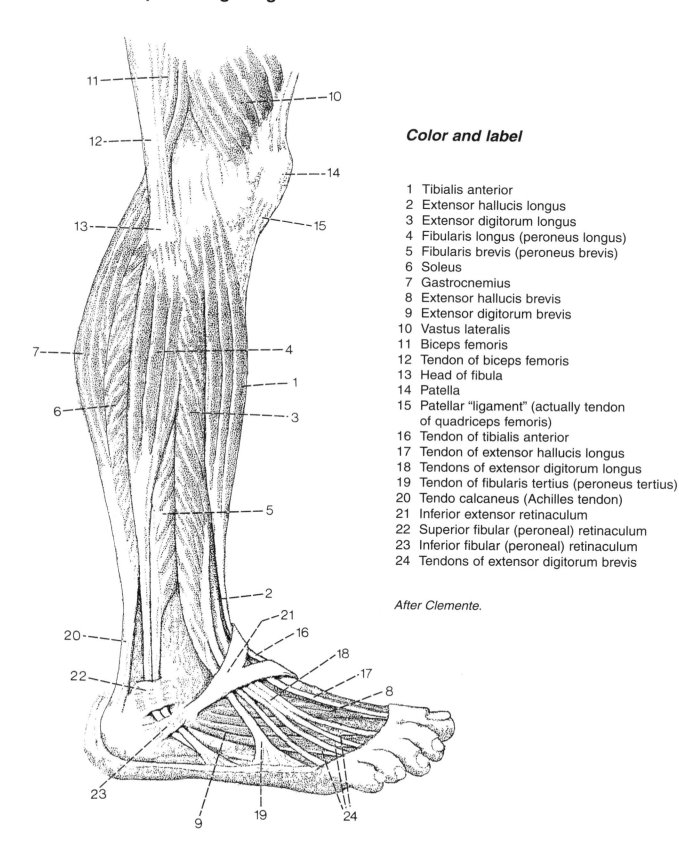

Color and label

1 Tibialis anterior
2 Extensor hallucis longus
3 Extensor digitorum longus
4 Fibularis longus (peroneus longus)
5 Fibularis brevis (peroneus brevis)
6 Soleus
7 Gastrocnemius
8 Extensor hallucis brevis
9 Extensor digitorum brevis
10 Vastus lateralis
11 Biceps femoris
12 Tendon of biceps femoris
13 Head of fibula
14 Patella
15 Patellar "ligament" (actually tendon
   of quadriceps femoris)
16 Tendon of tibialis anterior
17 Tendon of extensor hallucis longus
18 Tendons of extensor digitorum longus
19 Tendon of fibularis tertius (peroneus tertius)
20 Tendo calcaneus (Achilles tendon)
21 Inferior extensor retinaculum
22 Superior fibular (peroneal) retinaculum
23 Inferior fibular (peroneal) retinaculum
24 Tendons of extensor digitorum brevis

After Clemente.

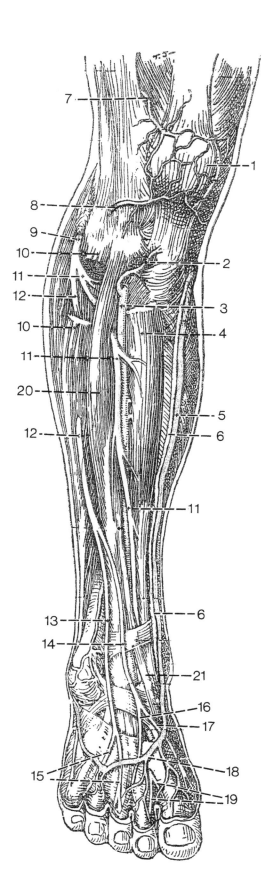

Color and label

1 Patella (knee cap); embedded in the tendon of the quadratus femoris: largest sesamoid bone in the body
2 Anterior recurrent tibial artery
3 Anterior tibial artery
4 Anterior tibialis muscle
5 Great saphenous vein
6 Saphenous nerve (branch of femoral nerve)
7 Superior lateral genicular artery
8 Inferior lateral genicular artery
9 Common peroneal (fibular) nerve
10 Peroneus (fibularis) longus muscle (section removed to show deep peroneal nerve)
11 Deep peroneal (fibular) nerve
12 Superficial peroneal (fibular) nerve
13 Intermediate dorsal cutaneus nerve
14 Medial dorsal cutaneus nerve
15 Dorsal cutaneus rami of superficial peroneal (fibular) nerve
16 Lateral branch of medial dorsal cutaneus nerve
17 Medial branch of medial dorsal cutaneus nerve
18 Dorsal venous arch of foot
19 Dorsal digital rami of deep peroneal (fibular) nerve; to adjacent skin between toes I and II
20 Extensor digitorum longus muscle
21 Tendon of extensor hallucis longus

Eycleshymer and Jones

47 Muscle attachments on the anterior leg*

Right leg

Color and label

1 Femur
2 Adductor tubercle and insertion of vertical part of adductor magnus
3 Lateral tibial condyle
4 Medial tibial condyle
5 Patella
6 Head of fibula
7 Lateral malleolus
8 Tibia
9 Tibial tuberosity
10 Medial malleolus
11 Talus

Color the origins (O) RED and the insertions (I) BLUE

12 Biceps femoris (I)
13 Peroneus longus (fibularis longus) (O)
14 Peroneus brevis (fibularis brevis) (O)
15 Extensor digitorum longus (O)
16 Extensor hallucis longus (O)
17 Tibialis posterior (O)
18 Iliotibial tract (I)
19 Tibialis anterior (O)
20 Quadriceps femoris (patellar "ligament") (I)
21 Sartorius (I)
22 Gracilis (I)
23 Semitendinosus (I)

*In anatomy the lower leg (from knee to ankle) is the leg, and the upper leg (from hip to knee) is the thigh.

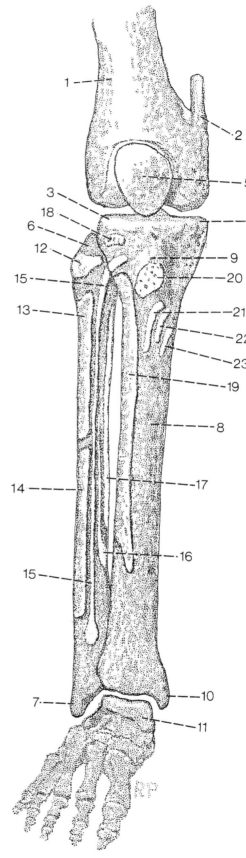

48 Muscle attachments on the posterior leg

Right leg

Label and color the origins (O) RED and the insertions (I) BLUE

1 Medial and lateral femoral condyles
2 Tendon of vertical part of adductor magnus (I)
3 Gastrocnemius (medial head) (O)
4 Gastrocnemius (lateral head) (O)
5 Intercondylar eminence
6 Medial tibial condyle
7 Lateral tibial condyle
8 Tibia
9 Fibula
10 Lateral malleolus
11 Medial malleolus
12 Head of fibula
13 Talus
14 Calcaneus
15 Semimembranosus (I)
16 Tibial collateral ligament
17 Popliteus (O)
18 Soleus (O)
19 Flexor digitorum longus (O)
20 Tibialis posterior (O)
21 Flexor hallucis longus (O)
22 Peroneus brevis (fibularis brevis) (O)
23 Biceps femoris (I)
24 Fibular collateral ligament
25 Popliteus (I)
26 Groove for tendon of flexor hallucis longus
27 Insertion of tendo calcaneus (gastrocnemius and soleus) (I)
28 Plantaris (O)

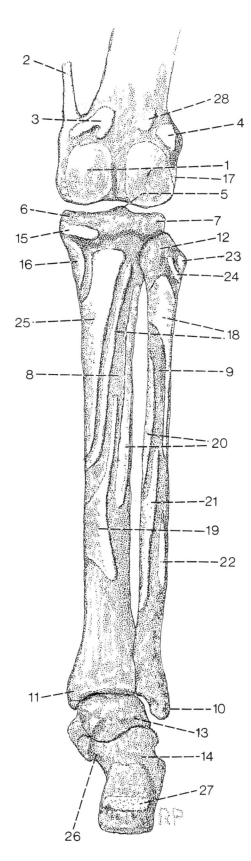

49 Bones of foot, medial aspect

Right foot

Color and label

1 Calcaneus
2 Talus
3 Navicular bone
4 Medial cuneiform bone
5 Intermediate cuneiform bone
6 First metatarsal bone
7 Proximal phalanx of big toe (hallux)
8 Distal phalanx of big toe
9 Sesamoid bones (in tendons of flexor hallucis brevis)
10 Medial malleolus (tibia)
11 Medial malleolar surface of talar trochlea
12 Tuberosity of calcaneus
13 Sustentaculum tali (of calcaneus)
14 Medial process of calcaneal tuberosity

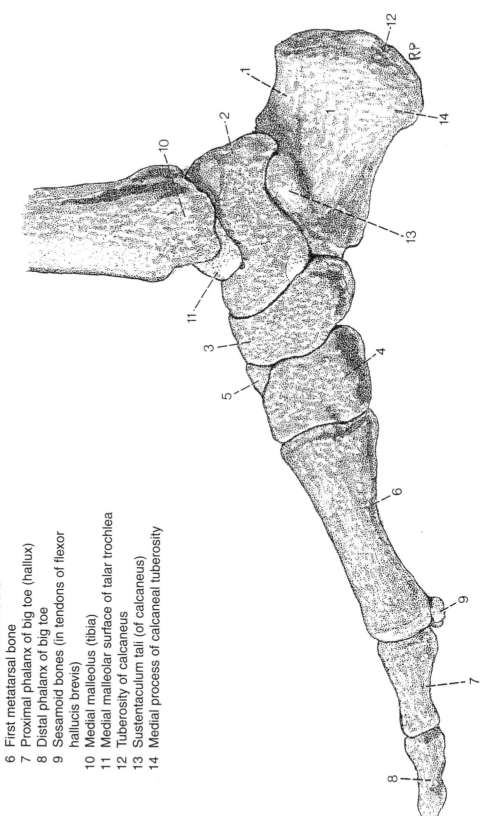

Plantar (inferior) aspect of the right foot

Color and label

1 Calcaneus (heel bone)
2 Calcaneal tuber (Latin, a
  swelling or protuberance)
3 Lateral process of
  calcaneal tuber
4 Medial process of
  calcaneal tuber
5 Sustentaculum tali
  (Latin, support of the talus)
6 Groove for the tendon of
  the flexor hallucis longus
  muscle
7 Head of talus (caput tali)
8 Cuboid bone
9 Tuberosity of cuboid bone
10 Navicular bone
11 Tuberosity of navicular bone
12 Medial cuneiform bone
13 Intermediate cuneiform bone
14 Lateral cuneiform bone
15 Tuberosity of first metatarsal bone
16 Groove for tendon of peroneus
  longus
17 Tuberosity of fifth metatarsal bone
18 Proximal phalanx of big toe
19 Distal phalanx of big toe;
  note that the big toe has
  only two phalanges
20 Medial and lateral sesamoid bones
21 Body of first metatarsal bone
  (of big toe or hallux)
22 Head of first metatarsal
23 Base of fifth metatarsal
24 Body of fifth metatarsal
25 Head of fifth metatarsal

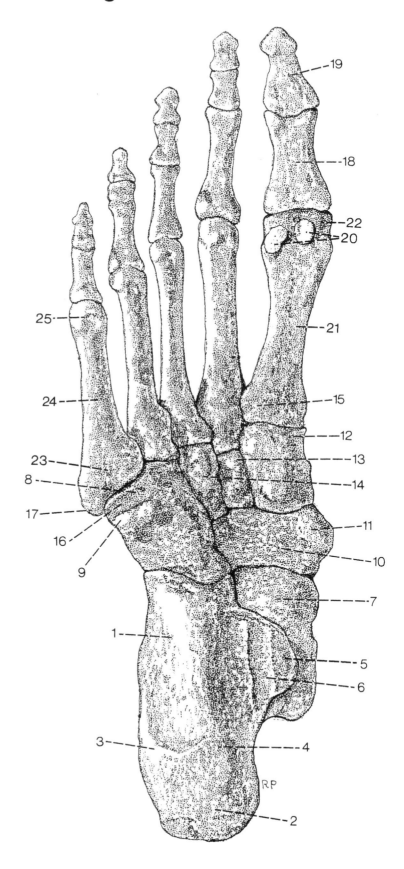

51 Plantar arteries

Right foot, plantar (inferior) aspect

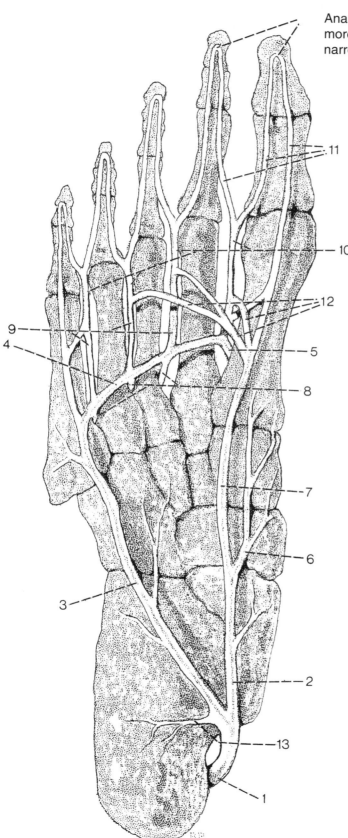

Anastomosing vessels are actually more numerous and much narrower than indicated here.

Color and label

1 Posterior tibial artery
2 Medial plantar artery
3 Lateral plantar artery
4 Deep plantar arch
5 Deep plantar artery (from dorsalis pedis artery)
6 Deep branch of medial plantar artery
7 Superficial branch of medial plantar artery
8 Perforating branches of plantar arch
9 Plantar metatarsal arteries
10 Common plantar digital arteries
11 Proper plantar digital arteries
12 Communicating branches
13 Calcaneal branch

After Hollinshead.

52 Plantar dissection of the right foot

Flexor digitorum brevis cut and largely removed

Color and label

1 Plantar aponeurosis (mainly lateral part)
2 Flexor digitorum brevis muscle (cut)
3 Lateral plantar artery (veins not shown)
4 Lateral plantar nerve
5 Abductor digiti minimi muscle
6 Quadratus plantae muscle
7 Deep (profundus) branch of
   lateral plantar nerve
8 Superficial branches of lateral
   plantar nerve
9 Flexor digiti minimi muscle
10 Plantar arch
11 Lumbrical muscles (arising
   on tendons of flexor
   digitorum longus)
12 Adductor hallucis
   (transverse head)
13 Tendons of flexor digitorum
   longus muscle
14 Tendons (cut) of flexor
   digitorum brevis
15 Fibrous tendon sheaths
16 Central part of plantar
   aponeurosis (cut)
17 Posterior tibial artery
18 Medial plantar artery
19 Medial plantar nerve
20 Abductor hallucis muscle (cut)
21 Tendon of flexor hallucis longus
22 Common plantar digital nerves
23 Flexor hallucis brevis muscle
24 Common plantar digital arteries
25 Proper plantar digital nerves
26 Proper plantar digital arteries

Redrawn from Tondury

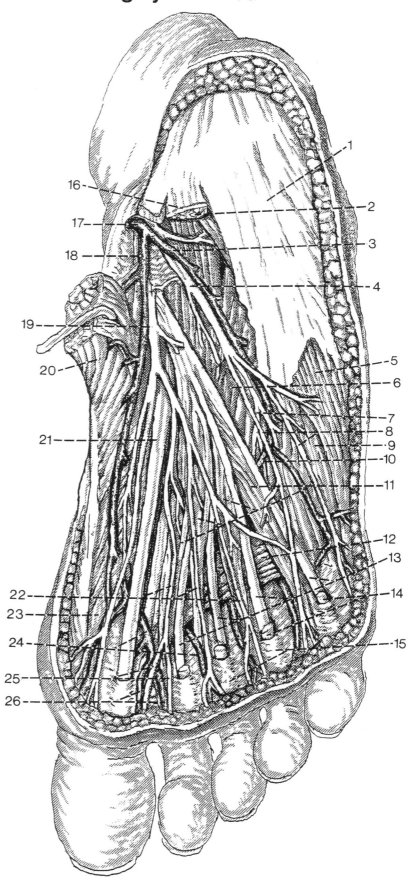

Viewed from behind

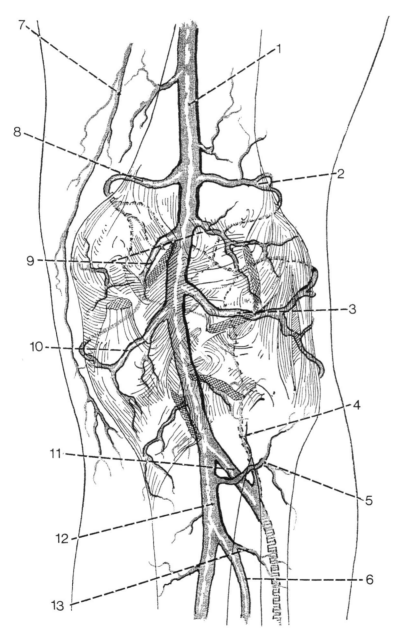

Eycleshymer and Jones

Color and label

1 Popliteal artery (a continuation of the femoral artery); note that the popliteal artery ends by dividing into the anterior and posterior tibial arteries
2 Lateral superior genicular artery
3 Lateral inferior genicular artery
4 Anterior recurrent tibial artery
5 Fibular branch
6 Fibular (peroneal) artery
7 Supreme genicular artery
8 Medial superior genicular artery
9 Sural arteries
10 Medial inferior genicular artery
11 Anterior tibial artery
12 Posterior tibial artery
13 Fibular nutrient artery (enters the bone)

Veins are not shown here. Veins accompanying the arteries (venae comitantes) have the same name as the artery and are often doubled (two veins accompany a single artery).

54 Arteries of the posterior leg

Right leg, posterior aspect

Color and label

1 Femoral artery
2 Popliteal artery
3 Descending genicular artery
4 Anterior tibial artery
5 Posterior tibial artery
6 Fibular (peroneal) artery
7 Lateral malleolar artery
8 Calcaneal artery
9 Lateral superior genicular artery
10 Medial superior genicular artery
11 Lateral inferior genicular artery
12 Medial inferior genicular artery
13 Anterior tibial recurrent artery
14 Fibular (peroneal) circumflex artery
15 Tibial collateral ligament
16 Fibular collateral ligament
17 Dorsalis pedis artery
   (seen through talis)
18 Interosseous membrane
19 Descending branch of lateral
   femoral circumflex artery

Not shown are the veins that accompany
the arteries (*venae comitantes*, Latin,
"veins that run with"). These are often doubled.

After Hollinshead

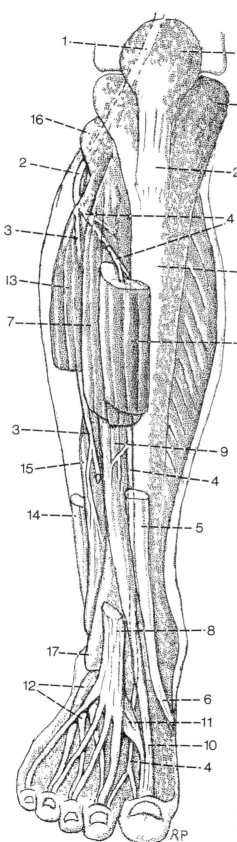

Color and label

1 Common fibular (peroneal) nerve (posterior to knee joint)
2 Common fibular (peroneal) nerve; external to neck of fibula. Note the exposed and vulnerable position of the common fibular nerve.*
3 Superficial fibular (peroneal) nerve; supplies fibularis (peroneus) longus and brevis; these two muscles evert (turn the sole outward) the foot
4 Deep fibular (peroneal) nerve; innervates the muscles of the anterior compartment: the extensor digitorum longus, the extensor hallucis longus, and the tibialis anterior; these muscles dorsiflex the foot (raise the foot up).
5 Tibialis anterior muscle
6 Tendon of tibialis anterior
7 Extensor digitorum longus muscle
8 Tendon of extensor digitorum
9 Extensor hallucis longus muscle
10 Tendon of extensor hallucis longus
11 Extensor hallucis brevis muscle
12 Extensor digitorum brevis muscle
13 Fibularis (peroneus) longus muscle
14 Tendon of fibularis longus
15 Fibularis (peroneus) brevis muscle
16 Head of fibula
17 Lateral malleolus
18 Patella (knee cap)
19 Tibia
20 Tibial tuberosity

*Damage to this nerve will result in **foot-drop**: in which the foot cannot be dorsiflexed (anterior compartment muscles paralyzed) nor everted (lateral compartment muscles paralyzed).

56 Foot: anterior-superior aspect

Left foot

Color and label

1 Tibia
2 Fibula
3 Interosseous membrane
4 Inferior extensor retinaculum
5 Medial malleolus
6 Lateral malleolus (and arterial rete from lateral malleolar artery)
7 Tibialis anterior muscle and tendon
8 Tendon of extensor hallucis longus
9 Extensor digitorum longus muscle
10 Tendon of extensor digitorum longus
11 Extensor hallucis brevis muscle
12 Extensor digitorum brevis muscle (number 3)
13 Deep fibular (peroneal) nerve
14 Anterior tibial artery
15 Abductor hallucis muscle
16 Fibularis (peroneus) brevis muscle
17 Fibularis (peroneus) longus muscle and tendon
18 Tibial nerve (divided) and posterior tibial artery and vein (also divided)
19 Superficial fibular (peroneal) nerve (divided)
20 Medial dorsal cutaneous branch of superficial fibular nerve
21 Intermediate dorsal cutaneous branch of superficial fibular nerve
22 Lateral dorsal cutaneous nerve (continuation of sural nerve)
23 Dorsal pedal digital nerves
24 Deep fibular (peroneal) nerve
25 Dorsal pedis artery (continuation of anterior tibial artery)
26 Dorsal digital nerves
27 First dorsal metatarsal artery
28 Lateral tarsal artery
29 Tendo calcaneus (Achilles tendon)
30 Soleus muscle
31 Tibialis posterior muscle
32 Flexor digitorum longus muscle
33 Flexor hallucis longus muscle

Based on and slightly modified from a Somso muscle

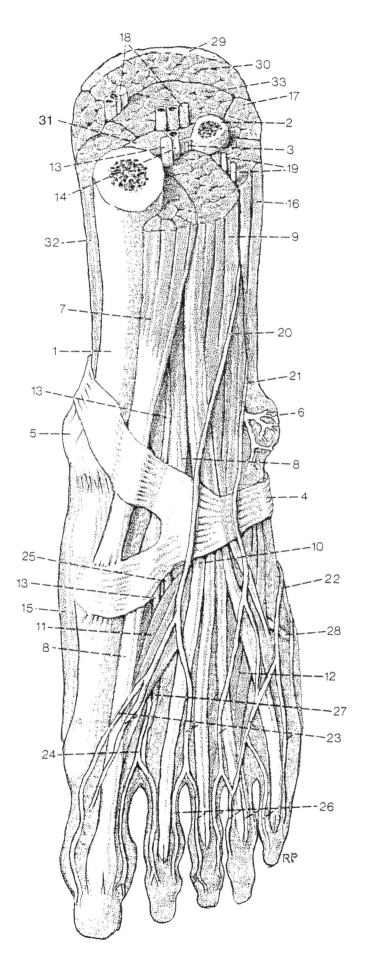

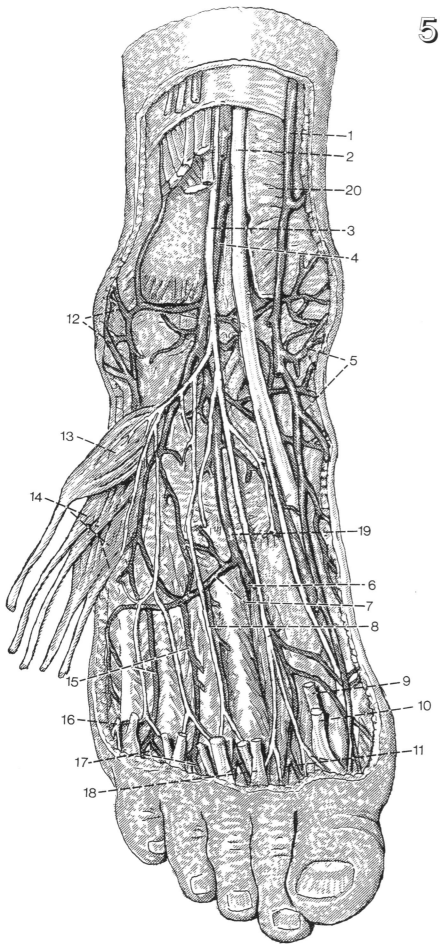

Deep dissection

Color and label

1 Great saphenous vein
2 Tendon of tibialis anterior muscle
3 Deep fibular (peroneal) nerve
4 Anterior tibial artery
5 Medial malleolar arterial and venous network (rete)
6 Deep plantar artery
7 Arcuate artery
8 Dorsal digital nerves
9 Tendon of extensor hallucis brevis (cut)
10 Tendon of extensor hallucis longus (cut)
11 Proper dorsal digital nerves
12 Lateral malleolar vascular plexus
13 Extensor hallucis brevis muscle (cut and pulled laterally)
14 Extensor digitorum brevis muscles (to toes 2-5)
15 Dorsal metatarsal arteries
16 Proper dorsal digital nerves
17 Dorsal digital arteries
18 Tendons of extensor digitorum longus (more superficial) and extensor digitorum brevis (deeper) to the second toe
19 Dorsalis pedis artery (continuation of anterior tibial artery)
20 Superior extensor retinaculum

Redrawn from Töndury

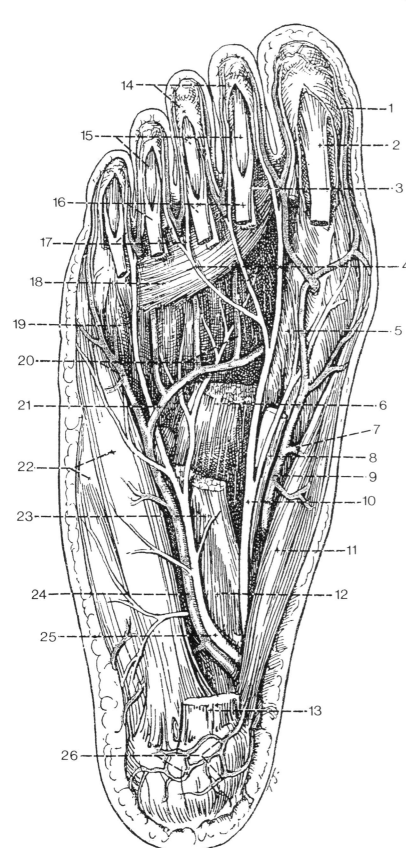

Color and label

1 Proper digital arteries and nerves
2 Flexor hallucis longus tendon
3 Common plantar digital artery
4 Common plantar digital nerves
5 Flexor hallucis brevis muscle
6 Adductor hallucis oblique head
7 Deep branch of medial plantar artery
8 Tendon of flexor hallucis longus (cut)
9 Medial plantar artery
10 Medial plantar nerve
11 Abductor hallucis muscle
12 Quadratus plantae muscle
13 Flexor digitorum brevis pedis muscle
14 Tendon sheaths (cut open)
15 Tendons of flexor digitorum longus
16 Tendons of flexor digitorum brevis
17 Proper plantar digital nerves
18 Adductor hallucis transverse head
19 Flexor digiti minimi muscle
20 Plantar metatarsal arteries
21 Plantar arch
22 Abductor digiti minimi muscle
23 Flexor digitorum longus muscle
24 Lateral plantar artery
25 Lateral plantar nerve
26 Calcaneal network

Eycleshymer and Jones

59 Plantar muscles I
And related structures of the left foot

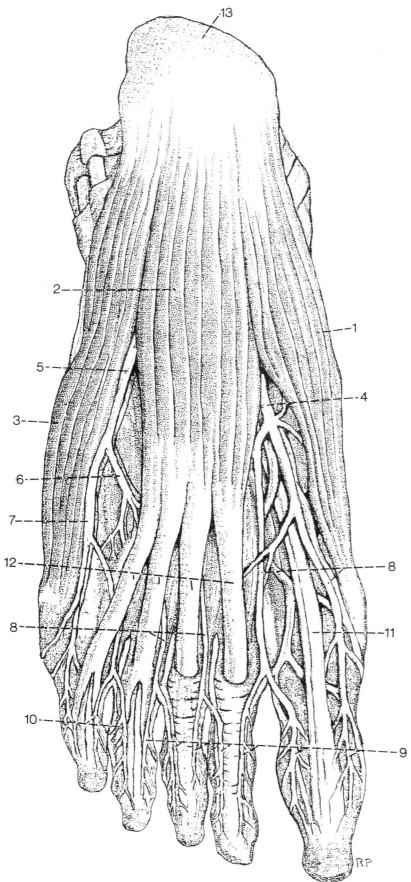

Color and label

1 Abductor hallucis*
2 Flexor digitorum brevis*
3 Abductor digiti minimi*
4 Medial plantar nerve; the tibial nerve ends by dividing into the medial plantar nerve and the lateral plantar nerve; the medial, the larger of the two plantar nerves, corresponds to the median nerve in the hand; it is accompanied by the medial plantar artery and vein (not shown).
5 Lateral plantar nerve; it corresponds to the ulnar nerve in the hand; it supplies the remaining 12 plantar muscles; it is accompanied by the lateral plantar artery and vein (not shown).
6 Deep branch of lateral plantar nerve
7 Superficial branch of lateral plantar nerve
8 Common plantar digital nerves
9 Proper plantar digital nerve (branches of medial plantar nerve)
10 Proper digital nerves (branches of lateral plantar nerve)
11 Tendon of flexor hallucis longus
12 Tendons of flexor digitorum brevis
13 Calcaneus

*Supplied by medial plantar nerve

Based on a Somso model

And related structures of the left foot

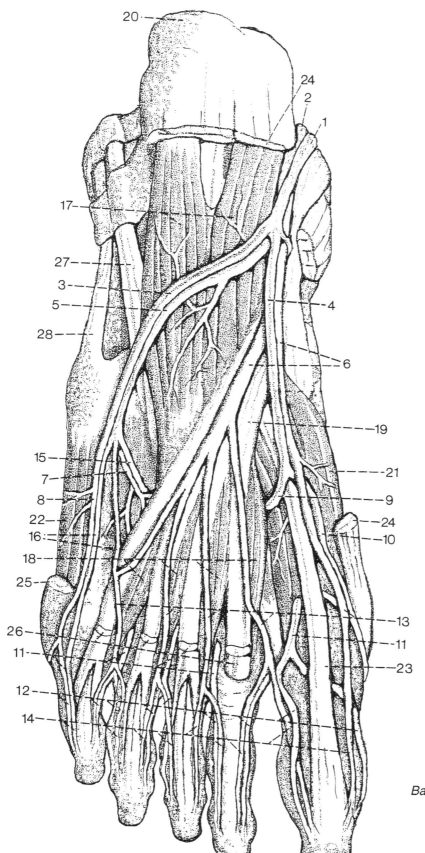

Color and label

1 Posterior tibial artery
2 Tibial nerve
3 Lateral plantar artery
4 Medial plantar artery
5 Lateral plantar nerve
6 Medial plantar nerve
7 Deep plantar arch
8 Superficial branch of
   lateral plantar artery
9 Deep branch of medial
   plantar artery
10 Superficial branch of
   medial plantar artery
11 Plantar metatarsal arteries
12 Proper plantar digital arteries
13 Common plantar digital nerves
14 Proper plantar digital nerves
15 Deep branch of lateral
   plantar nerve
16 Superficial branches of
   lateral plantar nerve
17 Quadratus plantae muscle*
18 Lumbrical muscles*
19 Tendon of flexor digitorum
   longus muscle*
20 Calcaneal tuberosity
21 Flexor hallucis brevis muscle
22 Flexor digiti minimi muscle
23 Tendon of flexor hallucis
   longus muscle
24 Abductor hallucis muscle
   (cut, origin and insertion only)
25 Abductor digiti minimi (cut)
26 Tendons (2-5) of flexor
   digitorum brevis (cut)
27 Tendon of peroneus (fibularis)
   longus muscle
28 Tendon of peroneus (fibularis)
   brevis inserting on tuberosity
   of fifth metatarsal

* Second layer of plantar muscles

Based on and modified from a Somso model

61 Plantar muscles III
And related structures of the left foot

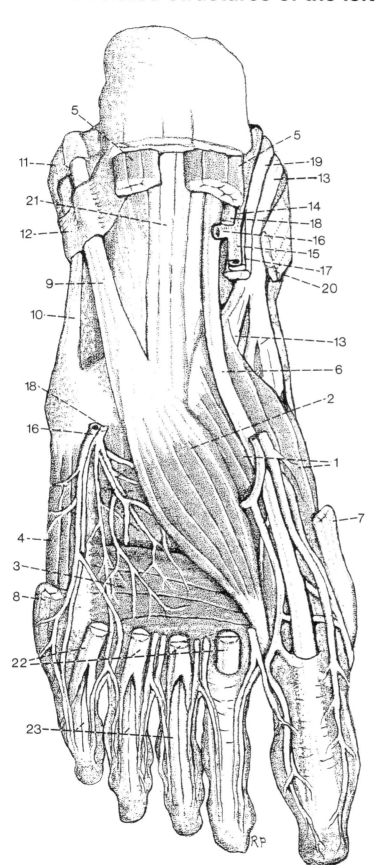

Color and label

1 Flexor hallucis brevis * muscle
2 Adductor hallucis * oblique head
3 Adductor hallucis * transverse head
4 Flexor digiti minimi *
5 Quadratus plantae (cut)
6 Tendon of flexor hallucis longus
7 Abductor hallucis (cut)
8 Abductor digiti minimi (cut)
9 Tendon of peroneus (fibularis) longus
10 Tendon of peroneus (fibularis) brevis
11 Superior fibular retinaculum
12 Inferior fibular retinaculum
13 Tendon of tibialis posterior
14 Posterior tibial artery
15 Medial plantar artery (cut)
16 Lateral plantar artery (cut)
17 Medial plantar nerve (cut)
18 Lateral plantar nerve (cut)
19 Tendon of flexor digitorum
    longus (cut)
20 Flexor retinaculum (cut)
21 Long plantar ligament
22 Four tendons of flexor
    digitorum brevis overlying
    (superficial to) four tendons
    of flexor digitorum longus (all
    8 tendons cut)
23 Tendons 3,4,5 of flexor
    digitorum longus passing through
    opened fibrous tendon sheaths
    to insert on terminal phalanges

* Third layer of plantar muscles
Based on a Somso model

62 Plantar muscles IV

And related structures of the left foot

Color and label

1 Tibial nerve
2 Posterior tibial artery
3 Medial plantar nerve
4 Lateral plantar nerve
5 Medial plantar artery
6 Lateral plantar artery
7 Superficial branch of
 medial plantar artery
8 Deep branch of
 medial plantar artery
9 Deep branch of
 lateral plantar nerve
10 Superficial branch of
 lateral plantar nerve
11 Deep branch of
 lateral plantar artery
 (deep plantar arch)
12 Superficial branch of
 lateral plantar artery
13 Plantar metatarsal arteries
14 Common plantar digital arteries
15 Proper plantar digital arteries
16 Common plantar digital nerves
17 Proper plantar digital nerves
 (note these are branches
 of the medial plantar nerve)
18 Plantar interosseous muscles;
 (*planta*, Latin, sole); fourth
 layer of plantar muscles;
 plantar flexion of the foot is
 flexion of the ankle that points
 the foot and toes downwards
19 Dorsal interosseous muscles
 fourth layer of plantar muscles;
 (the dorsum of the foot is the
 superior surface); dorsiflexion
 of the foot is the flexion of the
 foot **upwards** as in walking
 on the heels.
20 Tendon of tibialis posterior muscle
21 Tendon of fibularis (peroneus)
 longus muscle

Based on a Somso model

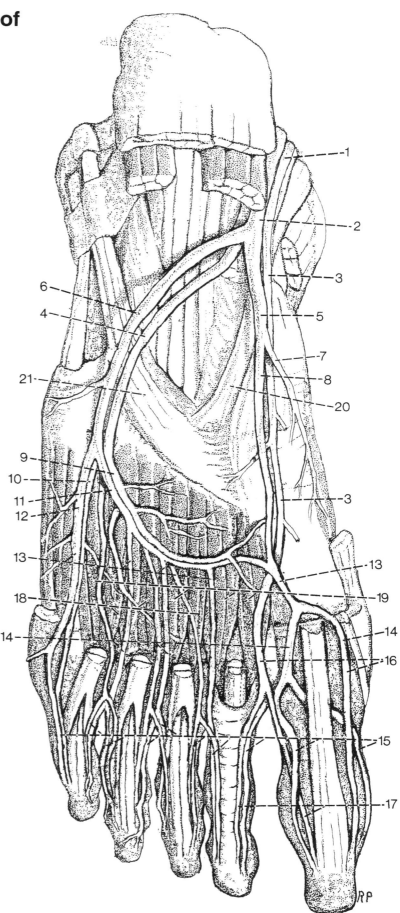

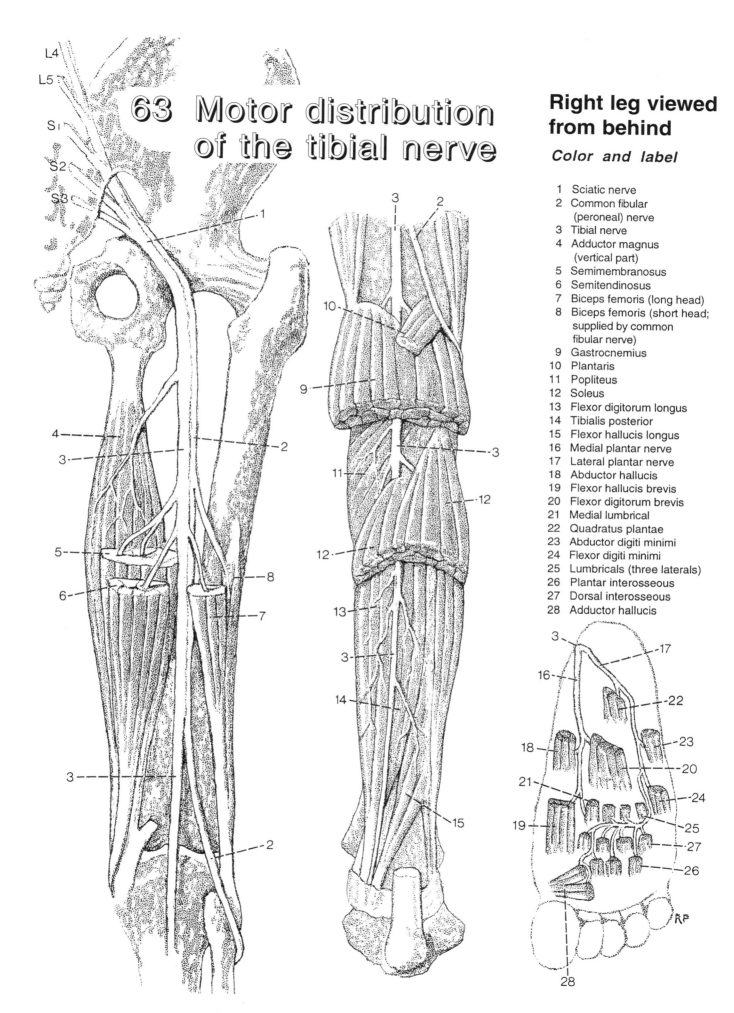

63 Motor distribution of the tibial nerve

Right leg viewed from behind

Color and label

1 Sciatic nerve
2 Common fibular (peroneal) nerve
3 Tibial nerve
4 Adductor magnus (vertical part)
5 Semimembranosus
6 Semitendinosus
7 Biceps femoris (long head)
8 Biceps femoris (short head; supplied by common fibular nerve)
9 Gastrocnemius
10 Plantaris
11 Popliteus
12 Soleus
13 Flexor digitorum longus
14 Tibialis posterior
15 Flexor hallucis longus
16 Medial plantar nerve
17 Lateral plantar nerve
18 Abductor hallucis
19 Flexor hallucis brevis
20 Flexor digitorum brevis
21 Medial lumbrical
22 Quadratus plantae
23 Abductor digiti minimi
24 Flexor digiti minimi
25 Lumbricals (three laterals)
26 Plantar interosseous
27 Dorsal interosseous
28 Adductor hallucis

64 Plantar arteries of the right foot

Viewed from below

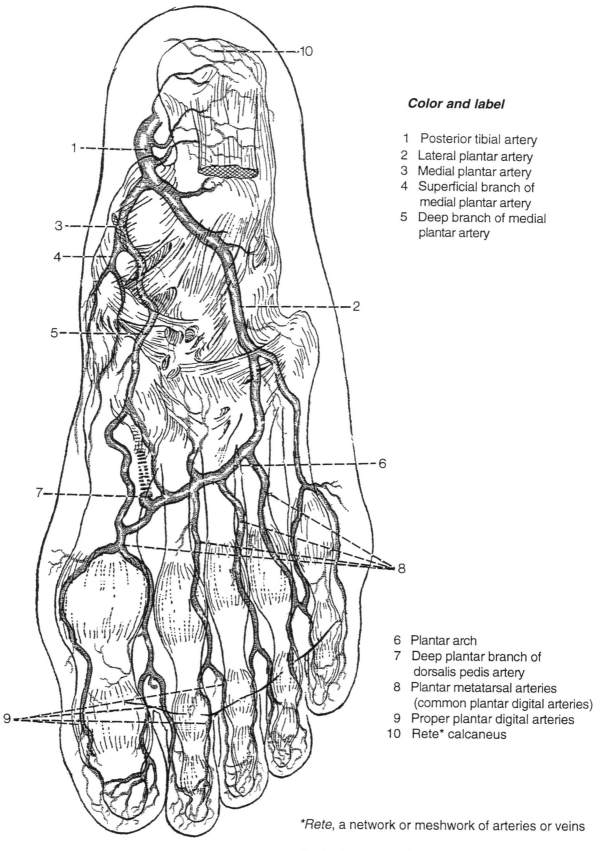

Color and label

1 Posterior tibial artery
2 Lateral plantar artery
3 Medial plantar artery
4 Superficial branch of
   medial plantar artery
5 Deep branch of medial
   plantar artery

6 Plantar arch
7 Deep plantar branch of
   dorsalis pedis artery
8 Plantar metatarsal arteries
   (common plantar digital arteries)
9 Proper plantar digital arteries
10 Rete* calcaneus

Rete, a network or meshwork of arteries or veins

Eycleshymer and Jones

65 Ligaments of the hip joint

Anterior view

Color and label

1 Anterior inferior iliac spine
2 Iliofemoral ligament
3 Greater trochanter
4 Lesser trochanter
5 Pubofemoral ligament
6 Obturator canal (opening in obturator membrane for obturator nerve artery and vein)
7 Obturator membrane
8 Ischiofemoral ligament (transverse band)
9 Ischiofemoral ligament (spiral band)
10 Neck of femur
11 Ischial tuberosity
12 Obturator foramen
13 Femur

Eycleshymer and Jones

Posterior view

RP

66 Frontal section of right hip joint

Viewed from the front

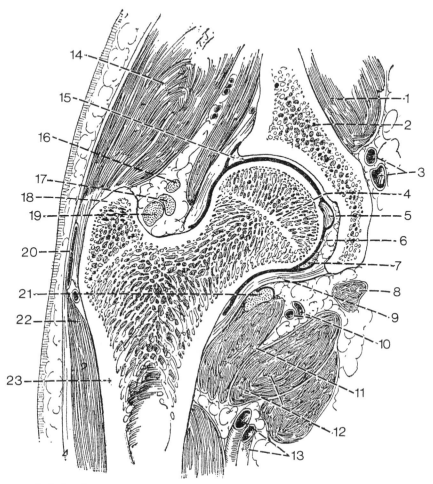

Color and label

1. Iliacus muscle
2. Pelvic bone (ilium)
3. External iliac artery and vein
4. Epiphyseal line in head of femur (remains of growth plate)
5. Ligament of head of femur; attached to fovea (pit) on the head of femur
6. Joint (articular) cavity
7. Transverse acetabular ligament; the acetabular labrum (15) bridges the acetabular notch as the transvers acetabular ligament, thereby forming a complete circle, which closely surrounds the head of the femur and helps hold it in place. (Clemente, 1985)
8. Obturator externus muscle
9. Joint (articular) capsule
10. Medial circumflex femoral artery and vein

11. Iliacus muscle
12. Pectineus muscle
13. Femoral artery and vein
14. Gluteus maximus muscle
15. Acetabular labrum (lip); a fibro-cartilaginous rim attached to the margin of the acetabulum, thereby deepening its cavity; it protects bony rim of the cup and smooths its surface. (Clemente, 1985)
16. Tendon of pyramidalis muscle
17. Obturator internus muscle
18. Greater trochanter
19. Obturator externus muscle
20. Bursa between greater trochanter and gluteus maximus
21. Tendon of psoas major
22. Vastus lateralis muscle
23. Femur

Eycleshymer and Jones

Viewed from in front
Knee is flexed in order to show cruciate ligaments

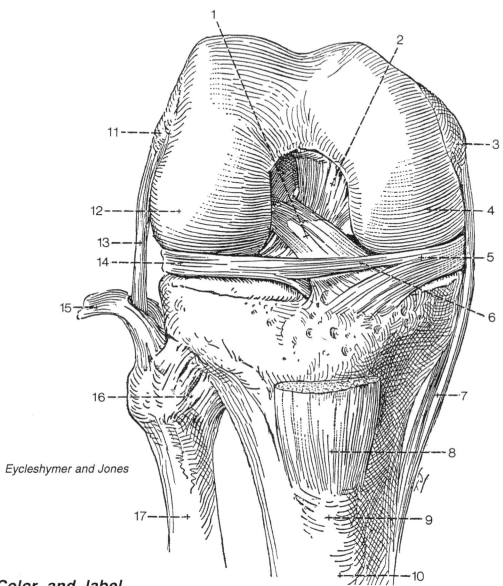

Eycleshymer and Jones

Color and label

1 Anterior cruciate ligament
2 Posterior cruciate ligament
3 Medial epicondyle of femur
4 Medial condyle of femur
5 Medial meniscus of knee joint; an oval crescent of fibrocartilage situated on the circumferential part of the medial superior articular surface of the tibia
6 Transverse ligament of knee; a fibrous cord of variable thickness connecting the anterior convex margin of the lateral meniscus to the anterior extremity of the medial meniscus (Churchill's Medical Dictionary)
7 Tibial collateral ligament

8 Patellar ligament; a continuation of the common tendon of the quadriceps femoris (cut); extends from the apex and inferior margins of the patella to insert on the tibial tuberosity
9 Tibial tuberosity
10 Tibia
11 Lateral epicondyle of femur
12 Lateral condyle of femur
13 Fibular collateral ligament
14 Lateral meniscus of knee joint; an oval crescent of fibrocartilage situated on the lateral superior articular surface of the tibia
15 Tendon of biceps femoris; inserting (mainly) on the head of the fibula
16 Anterior ligament of head of fibula
17 Fibula

Viewed from behind
Capsule has been removed

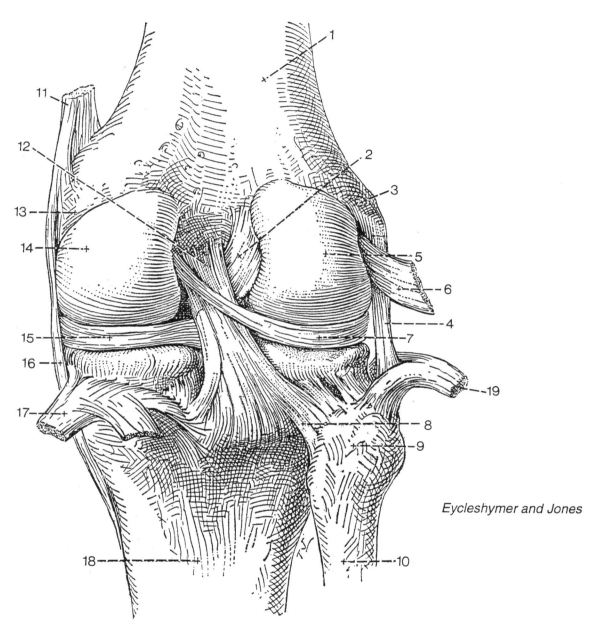

Eycleshymer and Jones

Color and label

1 Femur
2 Anterior cruciate ligament
3 Lateral epicondyle of femur
4 Fibular collateral ligament
5 Lateral condyle of femur
6 Popliteus muscle (cut)
7 Lateral meniscus
8 Posterior ligament of fibular head
9 Head of fibula

10 Fibula
11 Adductor magnus muscle (cut; vertical part)
12 Posterior cruciate ligament
13 Medial epicondyle of femur
14 Medial condyle of femur
15 Medial meniscus
16 Tibial collateral ligament
17 Semimembranosus muscle (cut)
18 Tibia
19 Biceps femoris muscle (cut)

69 Right knee joint

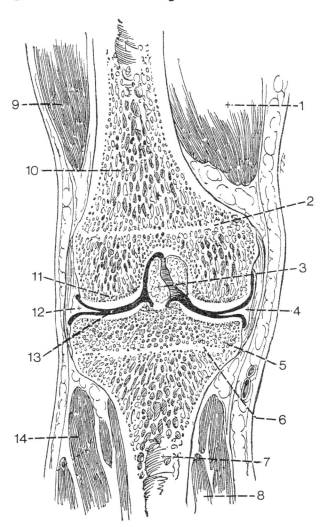

Figure A
Sectioned frontally
Viewed from the front

Color and label

1 Vastus medialis muscle
2 Epiphyseal line of femur
   (remains of growth plate)
3 Anterior cruciate ligament
4 Medial meniscus
5 Medial condyle of tibia
6 Epiphyseal line of tibia
   (remains of growth plate)
7 Tibia (shaft)
8 Gastrocnemius (medial head)
9 Vastus lateralis muscle
10 Femur (shaft)
11 Lateral femoral condyle
12 Lateral meniscus
13 Joint cavity
14 Gastrocnemius (lateral head)

Figure B
Superior articular
surface of tibia
Viewed from above

Color and label

1 Anterior cruciate ligament
2 Lateral meniscus
3 Posterior cruciate ligament
4 Medial meniscus
5 Transverse ligament of knee
6 Tibial tuberosity

Eycleshymer and Jones

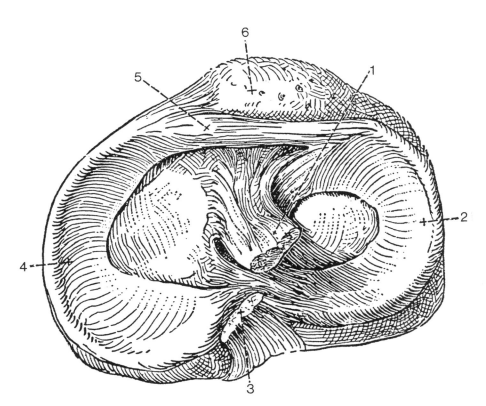

70 Muscle attachments on the dorsum of the foot

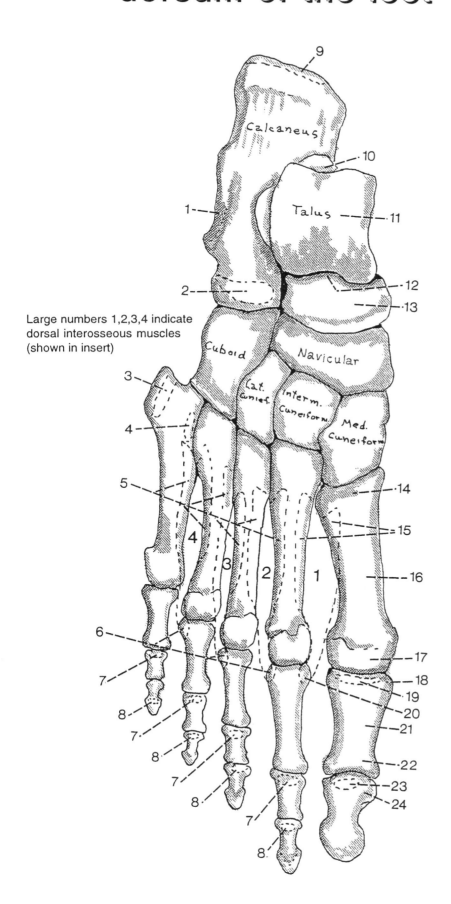

Large numbers 1,2,3,4 indicate
dorsal interosseous muscles
(shown in insert)

Color and label

(origins red; insertions blue)

1 Groove for tendon of peroneus
  brevis (fibularis brevis)
2 Origin of extensor digitorum brevis
3 Insertion of peroneus brevis
  (fibularis brevis)
4 Insertion of peroneus tertius
  (fibularis tertius)
5 Origins of dorsal interossei 2,3,4
6 Insertions of dorsal interossei 2,3,4
7 Insertion of extensor digitorum brevis
8 Insertion of extensor digitorum longus
9 Insertion of calcaneal tendon
10 Groove for tendon of
   flexor hallucis longus
11 Trochlea (Latin, pulley) of talus
12 Neck of talus
13 Head of talus
14 Base of first metatarsal
15 Origin of first dorsal interosseous
16 Body of first metatarsal
17 Head of first metatarsal
18 Base of proximal phalanx of big toe
19 Insertion of extensor hallucis brevis
20 Insertion of first dorsal interosseous
21 Body of proximal phalanx of big toe
22 Head of proximal phalanx of big toe
23 Insertion of extensor hallucis longus
24 Base of distal phalanx of big toe

After Clemente 1985

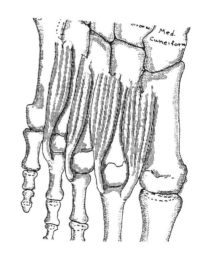

71 Muscle attachments on plantar surface of right foot

Color and label

(Origins red; insertions blue)

1 Origin of flexor digitorum brevis and abductor digiti minimi
2 Origin of quadratus plantae (lateral head)
3 Origin of quadratus plantae (medial head)
4 Insertion of tibialis posterior
5 Origin of flexor hallucis brevis
6 Groove for tendon of peroneus longus
7 Origin of flexor digiti minimi
8 Insertion of tibialis posterior
9 Insertion of tibialis posterior
10 Origins of plantar interossei 1,2,3
11 Insertion of flexor digiti minimi and abductor digiti minimi
12 Insertion of plantar interossei 1,2,3
13 Insertions of flexor digitorum brevis1,2,3,4
14 Insertion of flexor digitorum longus 1,2,3,4
15 Insertion of flexor hallucis longus
16 Insertion of adductor hallucis and flexor hallucis brevis
17 Insertion of flexor hallucis brevis and abductor hallucis
18 Sesamoid bones
19 Insertion of peroneus (fibularis) longus
20 Insertion of tibialis anterior
21 Origin of abductor hallucis

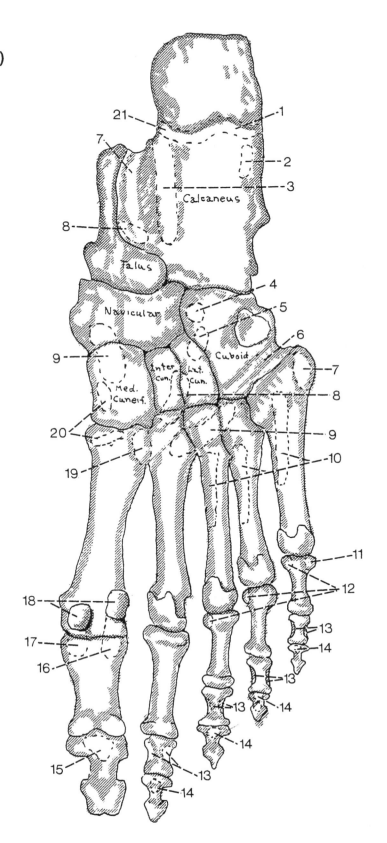

Pedigree (etymological cartoon)

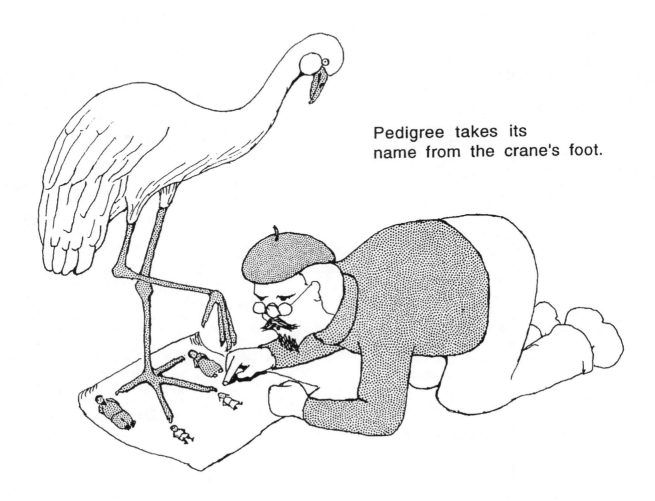

Pedigree takes its
name from the crane's foot.

Wilfred Funk points out that the word for one's bloodline or one's **pedigree** involves the **crane. Pedigree** is derived from the Latin "foot of the crane" (*pes, pedi*, "foot" + *de*, "of" + *grue*, "crane."). This came about because of the resemblance of a crane's foot to the lines of succession on a genealogical chart. So instead of saying "my family lineage looks like this," one would say "my family's *ped de grue* (foot of the crane) looks like this."

72 Muscles of plantar foot

Right foot inferior aspect

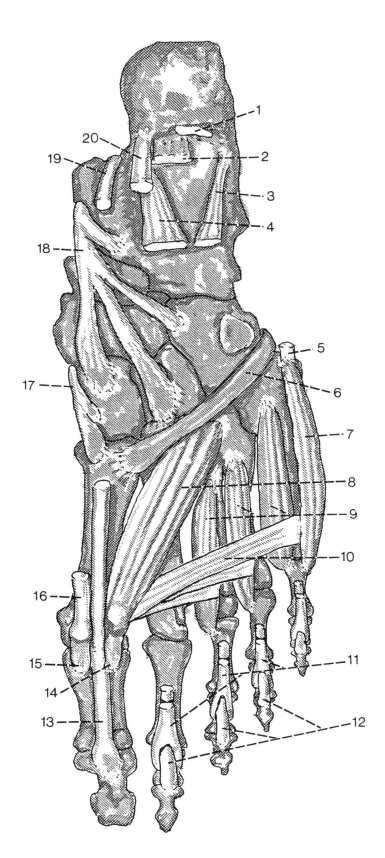

Color and label

1 Origin of flexor digitorum brevis
2 Abductor digiti minimi
3 Quadratus plantae (lateral head)
4 Quadratus plantae (medial head)
5 Insertion of abductor digiti minimi on tuberosity of 5th metatarsal
6 Tendon of peroneus (fibularis) longus
7 Flexor digiti minimi
8 Adductor hallucis (oblique head)
9 Plantar interossei (1st, 2nd, 3rd)
10 Adductor hallucis (transverse head)
11 Tendons (cut) of flexor digitorum brevis to toes 2,3,4
12 Tendons(cut) of flexor digitorum longus to toes 2,3,4
13 Tendon of flexor hallucis longus
14 Insertion of adductor hallucis (and flexor hallucis brevis)
15 Insertion of flexor hallucis brevis
16 Tendon of flexor hallucis brevis and abductor hallucis
17 Tendon of tibialis anterior
18 Tendon of tibialis posterior
19 Tendon of flexor hallucis longus
20 Origin of abductor hallucis

73 Planes of sections of right foot

Color and label

1 Calcaneus
2 Talus
3 Navicular bone
4 Medial cuneiform bone
5 Intermediate cuneiform bone
6 First metatarsal bone
7 Proximal phalanx of big toe (hallux)
8 Distal phalanx of big toe
9 Sesamoid bones (in tendons of flexor
   hallucis brevis)
10 Medial malleolus (tibia)
11 Medial malleolar surface of talar trochlea
12 Tuberosity of calcaneus
13 Sustentaculum tali (of calcaneus)
14 Medial process of calcaneal
   tuberosity

Bones of right foot medial aspect Sectioned through talus and calcaneus

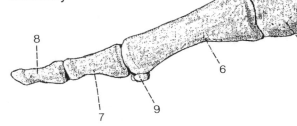

Sectioned through bases of metatarsal bones

Bones of right foot superior aspect

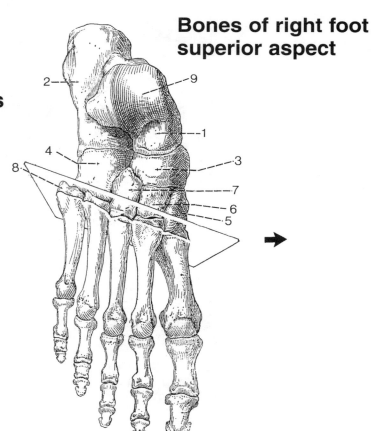

Bones of the right foot

Color and label

1 Talus
2 Calcaneus
3 Navicular
4 Cuboid
5 Medial cuneiform
6 Intermediate cuneiform
7 Lateral cuneiform
8 Tuberosity on base of 5th metatarsal
9 Trochlea of talus

Eycleshymer and Jones

Looking up from below

Color and label

1 Talus
2 Tendon of extensor hallucis longus
3 Tendon of tibialis anterior
4 Great saphenous vein
5 Talocalcaneal joint
6 Tendon of tibialis posterior ("Tom")
7 Sustentaculum tali (part of calcaneus)
8 Tendon of flexor digitorum longus ("Dick")
9 Tendon of flexor hallucis longus ("Harry")
10 Medial plantar artery, vein, and nerve
11 Lateral plantar artery, vein, and nerve
12 Quadratus plantae muscle
   (also called flexor accessorius)
13 Calcaneal tuberosity
14 Tendo calcaneus (Achilles tendon)
15 Calcaneus
16 Tendon of peroneus longus
17 Tendon of peroneus brevis
18 Talus, lateral tuberosity (or process)
19 Talocalcaneal joint
20 Extensor digitorum brevis muscle
21 Tendons of extensor digitorum longus
22 Dorsalis pedis artery (continuation
   of anterior tibial artery)
23 Interosseous talocalcaneal
   ligament in tarsal sinus

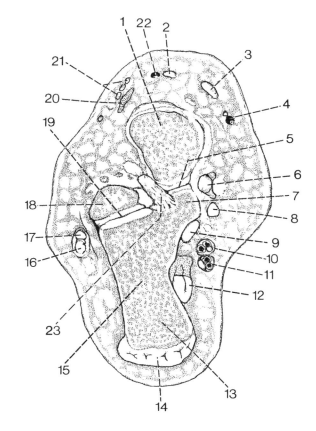

Viewed from the front

Color and label

1 Fifth metatarsal bone
2 Fourth metatarsal bone
3 Third metatarsal bone and
   interosseous ligament
4 Extensor digitorum brevis muscle
5 Lateral cuneiform (a small piece)
6 Tendon of extensor digitorum longus
7 Second metatarsal bone and
   interosseous ligament
8 Extensor hallucis brevis muscle
9 Medial cuneiform bone
10 Tendon of extensor hallucis longus
11 First metatarsal bone
12 Tendon of peroneus longus
13 Abductor hallucis muscle
14 Adductor hallucis muscle, oblique head
15 Flexor hallucis brevis muscle
16 Tendon of flexor hallucis longus
17 Medial plantar artery, vein, and nerve
18 Plantar aponeurosis
19 Flexor digitorum brevis muscle and tendons
20 Tendons of flexor digitorum longus muscle
21 Second plantar interosseous muscle and lateral
   plantar artery, vein, and nerve
22 Third plantar interosseous muscle
23 Flexor digiti minimi muscle
24 Opponens digiti minimi muscle
25 Abductor digiti minimi muscle

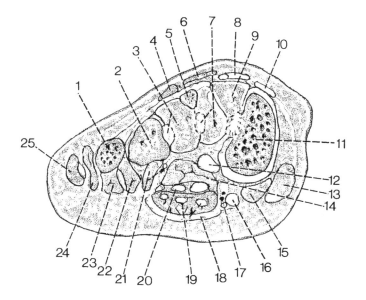

75 Ligaments of right ankle joint and foot

Viewed from the medial side

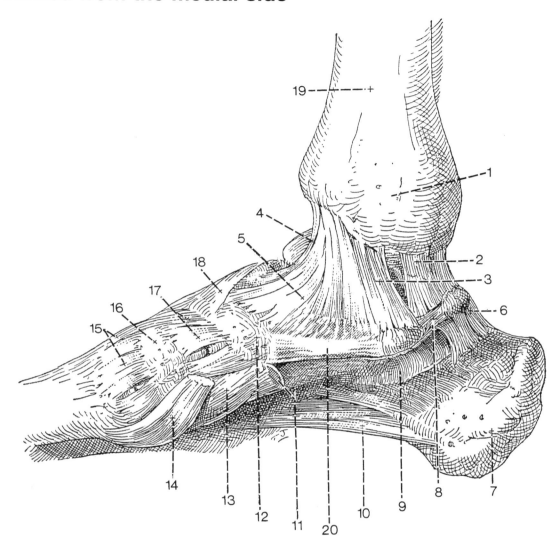

Color and label

1 Medial malleolus
2 Posterior tibiotalar ligament
  (part of deltoid ligament)
3 Tibiocalcaneal ligament
  (part of deltoid ligament)
4 Anterior tibiotalar ligament
  (part of deltoid ligament)
5 Tibionavicular ligament
  (part of deltoid ligament)
6 Posterior talocalcaneal ligament
7 Calcaneus
8 Medial talocalcaneal ligament
9 Groove for tendon of flexor
  hallucis longus muscle

10 Long plantar ligament
11 Tendon of tibialis posterior muscle
12 Navicular bone
13 Plantar cuneonavicular ligament
14 Tendon of tibialis anterior
15 Dorsal tarsometatarsal ligaments
16 Cunieform bone
17 Dorsal cuneonavicular ligament
18 Talonavicular ligament
19 Tibia
20 Plantar calcaneonavicular ligament

Eycleshymer and Jones

Right foot lateral view

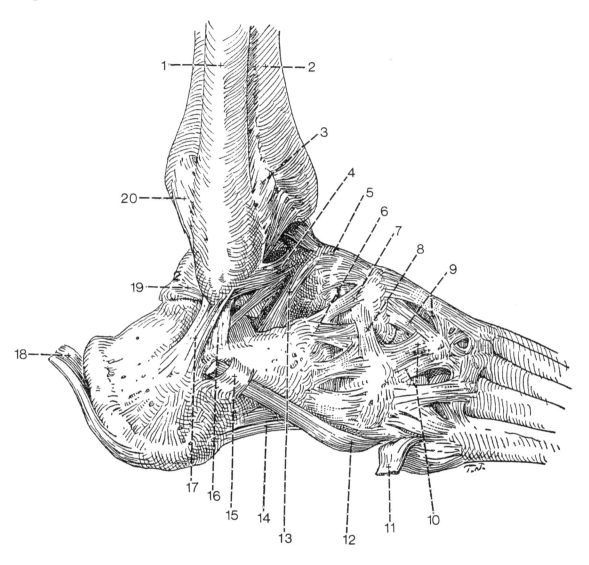

Color and label

1 Fibula
2 Tibia
3 Anterior tibiofibular ligament
4 Anterior talofibular ligament
5 Talonavicular ligament
6 Calcaneocuboid ligament
  (part of bifurcated ligament)
7 Calcaneonavicular ligament
  (part of bifurcated ligament)
8 Dorsal cuboideonavicular ligament
9 Dorsal cuneonavicular ligaments

10 Dorsal cuneocuboid ligaments
11 Tendon of fibularis (peroneus) brevis
12 Tendon of fibularis (peroneus) longus
13 Anterior talocalcaneal ligament
14 Long plantar ligament
15 Inferior fibular (peroneal) retinaculum
16 Lateral talocalcaneal ligament
17 Calcaneofibular ligament
18 Calcaneal tendon
19 Posterior talofibular ligament
20 Posterior tibiofibular ligament

Eycleshymer and Jones with modification

Right foot viewed from behind

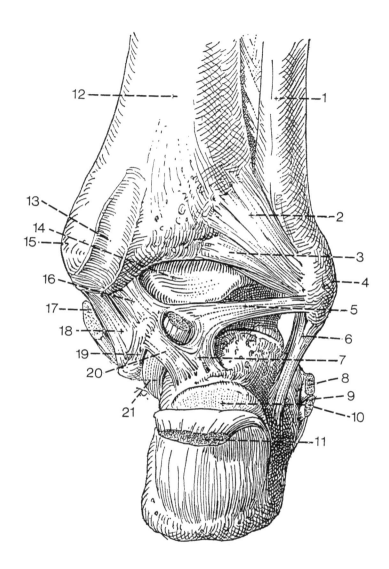

Color and label

1 Fibula
2 Posterior tibiofibular ligament
3 Inferior transverse
(tibiofibular) ligament
4 Lateral malleolus
5 Posterior talofibular ligament
6 Calcaneofibular ligament
7 Talocalcaneal ligament
8 Tendon of peroneus
(fibularis) brevis
9 Tendon of peroneus
(fibularis) longus
10 Calcaneus (tuberosity)
11 Tendon calcaneus (Achilles)
(cut and pulled posterior)
12 Tibia

13 Groove for tendon of tibialis posterior
14 Trochlea (pulley, Latin) of talus
15 Medial malleolus
16 Posterior tibiotalar ligament
(part of deltoid ligament)
17 Tendon of tibialis posterior
("**Tom**" of "Tom, Dick, and Harry")
18 Tibiocalcaneal ligament
(part of deltoid ligament)
19 Medial talocalcaneal ligament
20 Retinaculum for tendon of flexor
hallucis longus
21 Tendon of flexor hallucis longus
("**Harry**" of "Tom, Dick, and Harry")

modified from Eycleshymer and Jones

Viewed from below

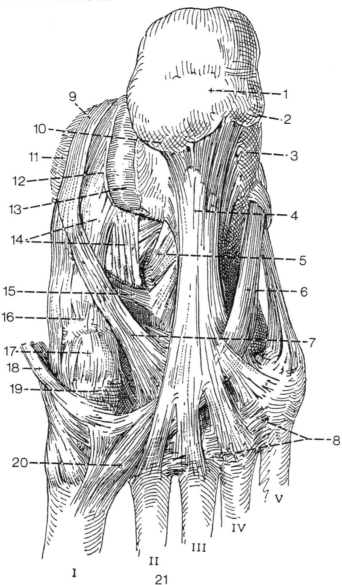

Color and label

1 Calcaneal tuberosity
2 Lateral process of calcaneal tuberosity
3 Calcaneus
4 Long plantar ligament
5 Plantar calcaneocuboid ligament
6 Tendon of peroneus (fibularis) longus muscle
7 Tendon of tibialis posterior muscle
8 Plantar intermetatarsal ligaments
9 Tendon of tibialis posterior muscle
10 Medial process of calcaneal tuberosity
11 Talus

12 Sustentaculum tali ("support for the talus"; shelf-like part of the calcaneus)
13 Sulcus (groove) on underside of sustentaculum tali for flexor hallucis longus tendon
14 Plantar calcaneonavicular ligament
15 Plantar cuboideonavicular ligament
16 Navicular bone
17 Plantar cuneonavicular ligament
18 Tibialis anterior tendon
19 Medial cuneiform bone
20 Peroneus (fibularis) longus tendon
21 Metatarsal bones

Eycleshymer and Jones with modification

79 Frontal section of ankle and foot

Right foot and ankle viewed from the front

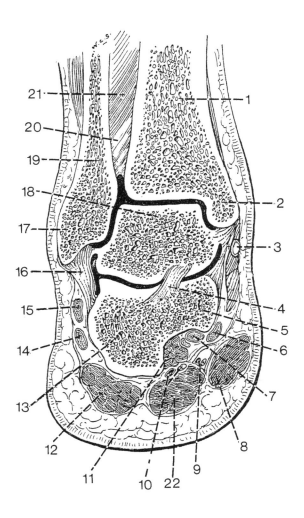

Color and label

1 Tibia
2 Medial malleolus
3 Tendon of tibialis posterior ("Tom")
4 Interosseous talocalcaneal ligament
5 Sustentaculum tali
6 Tendon of flexor digitorum longus ("Dick")
7 Tendon of flexor hallucis longus ("Harry")
8 Abductor hallucis muscle
9 Medial plantar nerve and artery (veins not shown)
10 Lateral plantar nerve and artery
11 Quadratus plantae muscle
12 Abductor digiti quinti muscle
13 Calcaneus
14 Tendon of peroneus (fibularis) longus
15 Tendon of peroneus (fibularis) brevis
16 Calcaneofibular ligament
17 Lateral malleolus
18 Talus
19 Fibula
20 Tibiofibular ligament
21 Interosseous membrane
22 Flexor digitorum brevis muscle

Color and label

1 Flexor hallucis longus muscle
2 Abductor hallucis longus muscle
3 Medial plantar nerve and artery
4 Flexor digitorum brevis muscle
5 Lateral plantar nerve and artery
6 Plantar aponeurosis
7 Plantar arch
8 Abductor digiti minimi muscle

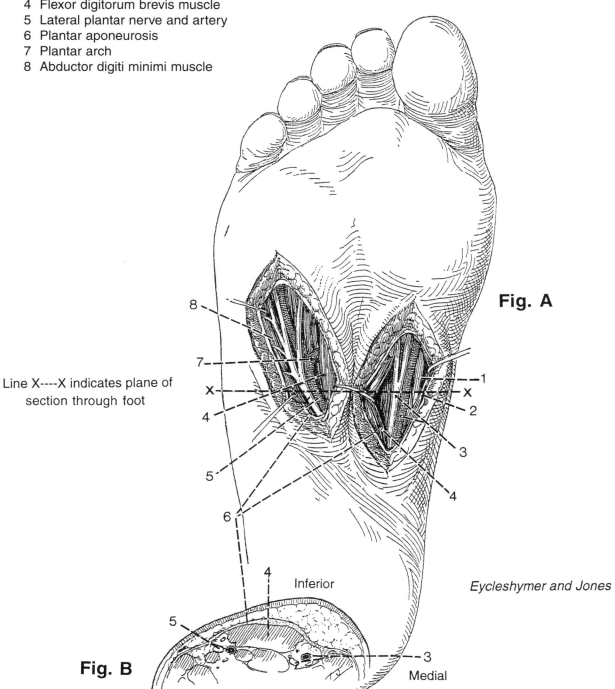

Fig. A

Line X----X indicates plane of
section through foot

Eycleshymer and Jones

Inferior

Fig. B

Lateral

Medial

Cross section of inferior foot

81 Incision in back of medial malleolus

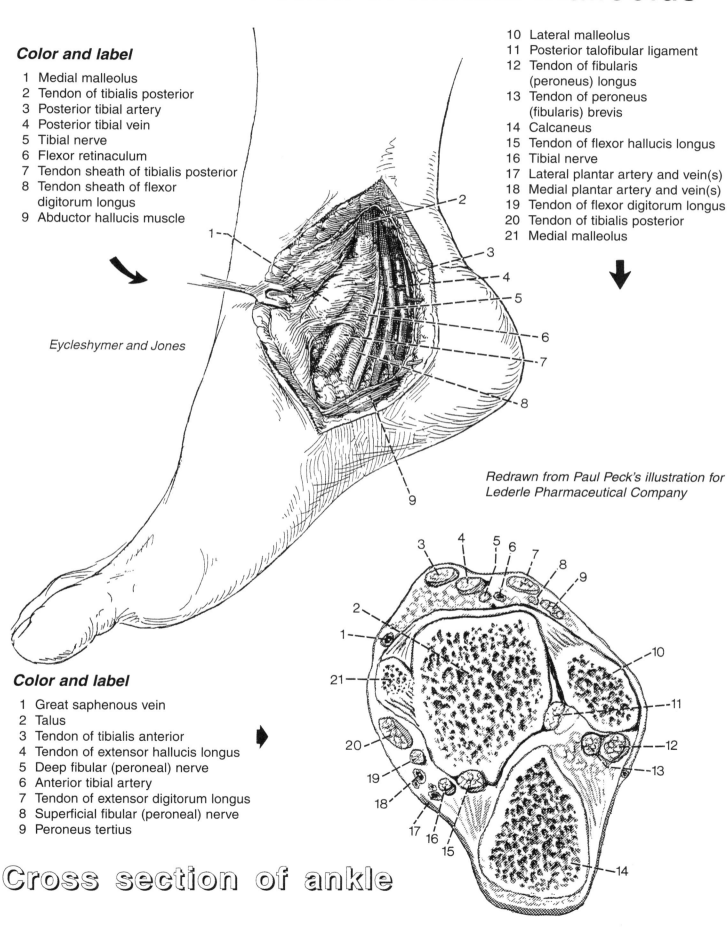

Color and label

1. Medial malleolus
2. Tendon of tibialis posterior
3. Posterior tibial artery
4. Posterior tibial vein
5. Tibial nerve
6. Flexor retinaculum
7. Tendon sheath of tibialis posterior
8. Tendon sheath of flexor digitorum longus
9. Abductor hallucis muscle

10. Lateral malleolus
11. Posterior talofibular ligament
12. Tendon of fibularis (peroneus) longus
13. Tendon of peroneus (fibularis) brevis
14. Calcaneus
15. Tendon of flexor hallucis longus
16. Tibial nerve
17. Lateral plantar artery and vein(s)
18. Medial plantar artery and vein(s)
19. Tendon of flexor digitorum longus
20. Tendon of tibialis posterior
21. Medial malleolus

Eycleshymer and Jones

Redrawn from Paul Peck's illustration for Lederle Pharmaceutical Company

Color and label

1. Great saphenous vein
2. Talus
3. Tendon of tibialis anterior
4. Tendon of extensor hallucis longus
5. Deep fibular (peroneal) nerve
6. Anterior tibial artery
7. Tendon of extensor digitorum longus
8. Superficial fibular (peroneal) nerve
9. Peroneus tertius

Cross section of ankle

82 Cutaneous nerves of the lower extremity

Anterior aspect

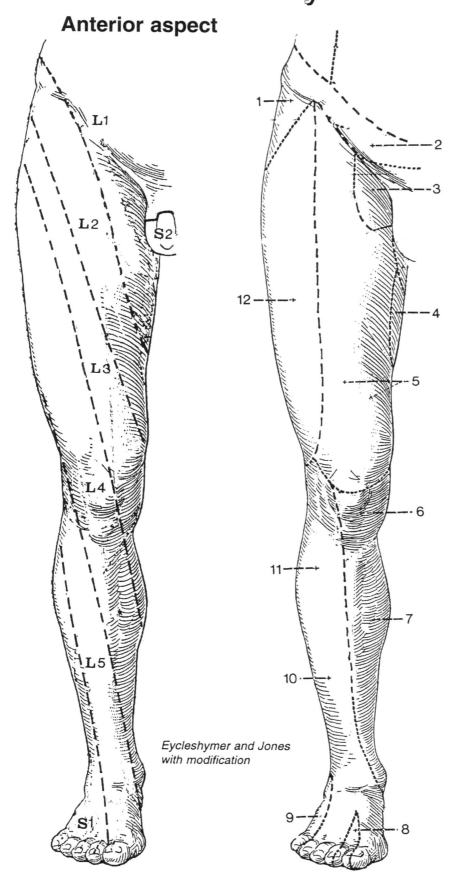

L1
L2
S2
L3
L4
L5
S1

1
2
3
12
4
5
6
11
7
10
9
8

Eycleshymer and Jones with modification

Letters and numbers in the left figure indicate the spinal origin of the nerves distributed to each area. The figure at the right shows the area of distribution of the cutaneous nerves.

Color and label

1 Lateral cutaneous ramus of subcostal nerve (T 12)
2 Anterior cutaneous ramus of iliohypogastric nerve
3 Ilioinguinal nerve
4 Obturator nerve
5 Anterior cutaneous ramus of femoral nerve
6 Infrapatellar ramus of saphenous nerve (branch of femoral nerve)
7 Saphenous nerve
8 Deep peroneal (fibular) nerve
9 Sural nerve
10 Superficial peroneal (fibular) nerve
11 Lateral sural cutaneous nerve
12 Lateral femoral cutaneous nerve

83 Cutaneous nerves of the lower extremity

Posterior aspect

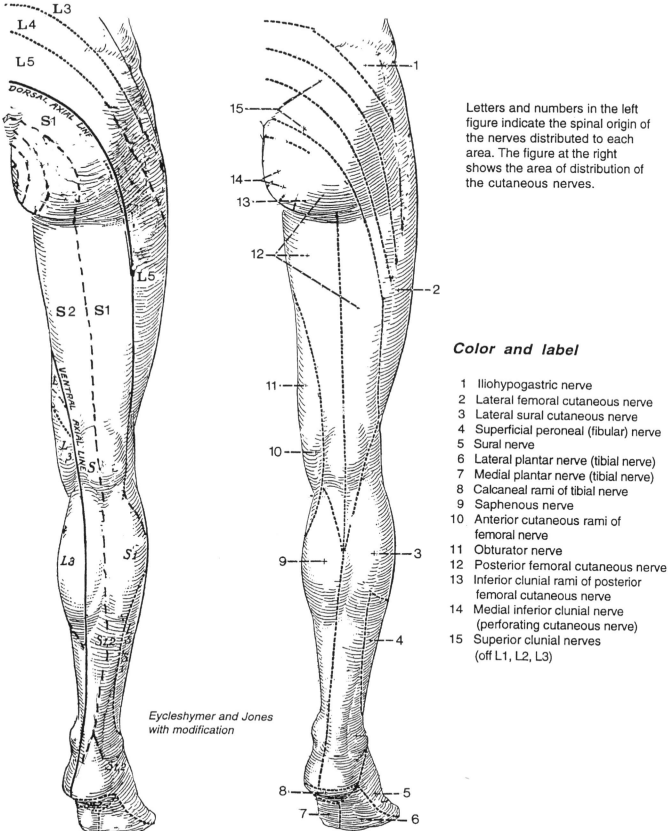

Letters and numbers in the left figure indicate the spinal origin of the nerves distributed to each area. The figure at the right shows the area of distribution of the cutaneous nerves.

Color and label

1 Iliohypogastric nerve
2 Lateral femoral cutaneous nerve
3 Lateral sural cutaneous nerve
4 Superficial peroneal (fibular) nerve
5 Sural nerve
6 Lateral plantar nerve (tibial nerve)
7 Medial plantar nerve (tibial nerve)
8 Calcaneal rami of tibial nerve
9 Saphenous nerve
10 Anterior cutaneous rami of femoral nerve
11 Obturator nerve
12 Posterior femoral cutaneous nerve
13 Inferior clunial rami of posterior femoral cutaneous nerve
14 Medial inferior clunial nerve (perforating cutaneous nerve)
15 Superior clunial nerves (off L1, L2, L3)

Eycleshymer and Jones with modification

Notes

Notes